Hygge

Master the Danish Art of Happiness to Bring Harmony and Balance in Your Life. Enjoy Coziness with Simple Things Improving Health, Relationships, Cooking and Home Decor

SUSANNE LAGOM

© **Copyright 2019 - All rights reserved.**

The content contained within this book may not be reproduced, duplicated or transmitted without direct written permission from the author or the publisher.

Under no circumstances will any blame or legal responsibility be held against the publisher, or author, for any damages, reparation, or monetary loss due to the information contained within this book. Either directly or indirectly.

Legal Notice:

This book is copyright protected. This book is only for personal use. You cannot amend, distribute, sell, use, quote or paraphrase any part, or the content within this book, without the consent of the author or publisher.

Disclaimer Notice:

Please note the information contained within this document is for educational and entertainment purposes only. All effort has been executed to present accurate, up to date, and reliable, complete information. No warranties of any kind are declared or implied. Readers acknowledge that the author is not engaging in the rendering of legal, financial, medical or professional advice. The content within this book has been derived from various sources. Please consult a licensed professional before attempting any techniques outlined in this book.

By reading this document, the reader agrees that under no circumstances is the author responsible for any losses, direct or indirect, which are incurred as a result of the use of information contained within this document, including, but not limited to, — errors, omissions, or inaccuracies.

Table of Contents

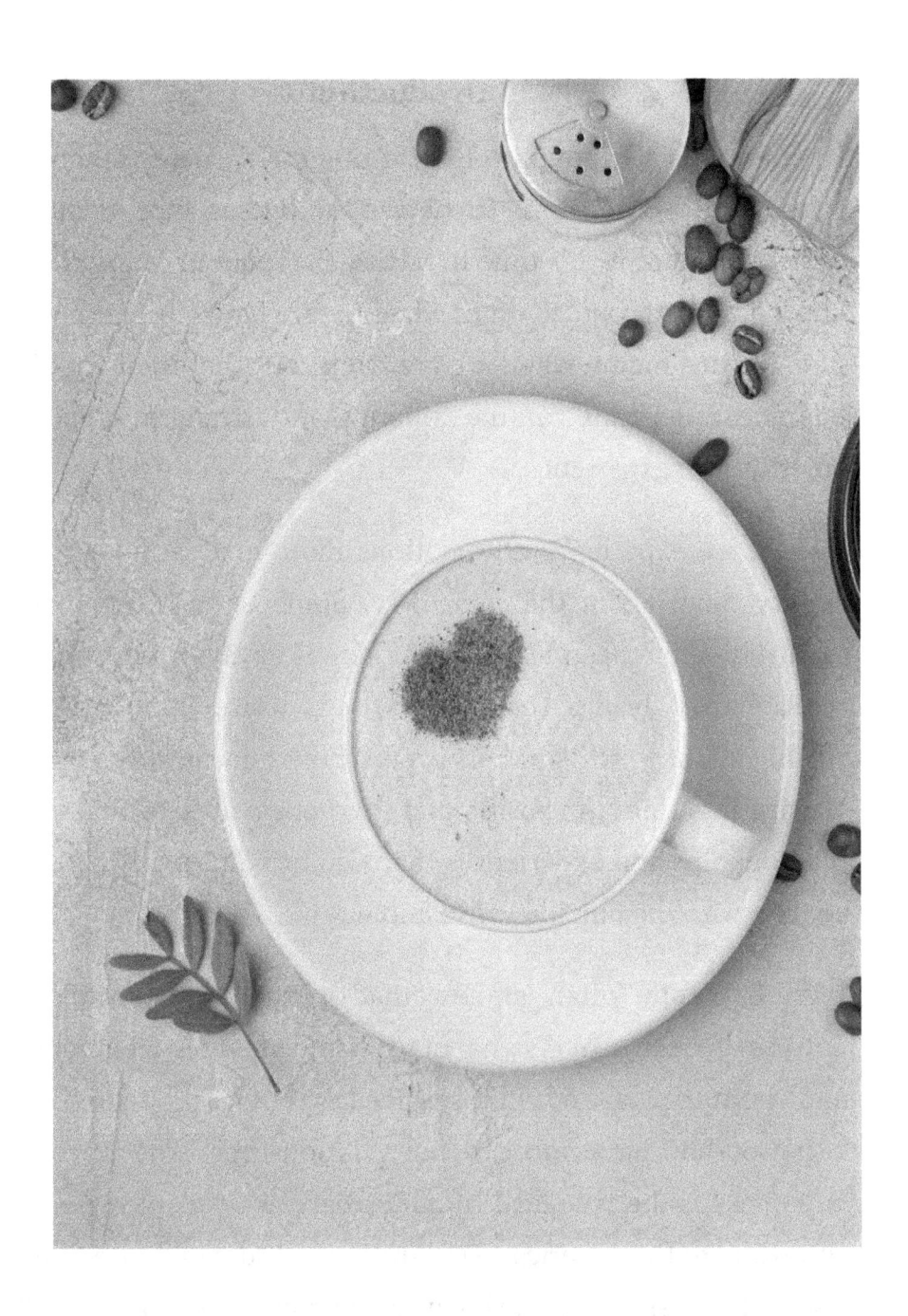

Introduction

Happiness is the potion; elixir of our life. It doesn't know the rules. That is freedom, frivolity. Our bodies hide it as if to protect it, but now it's time to release it sooner or later. We each know how to recognize times when we are happy because we are not. We are happy when we are calm, but the intensity of our happiness depends on the amount and strength of positive emotions we experience.

In fact, we experience all emotions more or less, but we don't convey them all in the same way. Some try to keep them to themselves, but even in this case there is always an unconscious reaction that brings them out. Others share it by talking or writing about it, while others even succeed in capturing it in art. We are in an era of sharing and everyone wants to find simple relationships and experiences that also bring us back to genuine contact with the outside world and nature.

Who is happy often smiles, that is the unmistakable and universally recognized signal of joy. Happy people feel more free and spontaneous, and, in a self-feeding circle, they are happier because they have more social relationships. The pursuit of happiness is the true goal of our society, even a universal right according to the American Declaration of Independence, but it is also a dimension that varies from person to person, as well as the ways of perceiving and demonstrating it.

Today the topic is truly succulent, more and more people are wondering what happiness is. Talking about happiness is always very difficult, as the concept itself of happiness is so personal and subjective that it is really complicated to understand where the border lies... Unfortunately, there are moments in life when experiencing happiness is not easy, you want a mourning that affects us closely, you want because we have lost your job, you want because the person we love has left us, and with the examples we could continue endlessly.

The important thing is that you can realize that they are "only" moments, and I think it is right to live them and go through that pain to the end, then let go, abandon them, and return to that underlying happiness that belongs to you and that must depend only and exclusively by yourself instead of being entrusted to external factors.

Hygge is a Swedish word which, according to some, would have the same root as the English word "Hug", which means hug. It is a lifestyle, a philosophy, a strategy for building lasting happiness. In this book learn how and why we should all live hygge. Especially in the winter season, when cold and lack of light intensify, many feel higher levels of anxiety and sadness, the Danish philosophy of life can be a valid help to reduce stress and better live the present. In the northern countries, winter seems endless, nature is often hostile and darkness falls for months. For this reason the house and everything that is emotionally related to it has taken on a fundamental meaning for the peoples who live near the Polo.

The house is placed at the center of daily happiness, it is a safe and comfortable environment, which becomes the gravitational center of everyday life. At home, much more often than outside, you are happy and safe. For this reason the Swedes, but more generally all the peoples of Northern Europe, pay particular attention to furnishing and caring for the home, which must be able to transmit beneficial sensations and ward off sadness and depression.

Although their winter is colder and longer, the Danes have been the happiest people in the world for over 40 years. Their secret seems to be in the lifestyle (hygge). Mental health is a topic that too often is overlooked or simply ignored by most individuals. For a long time it was taboo in the world to talk about your own psychological problems or even to solve them with psychological therapy. Fortunately, things have changed, but there is still a long way to go to spread the idea that mental well-being is as important as physical well-being.

While the community is waiting for change, everyone can (and must) learn to take care of their mental health in a small way.

Hygge is the perfect tool to start from home in a few small steps. We all live under pressure, forced to do many things at the same time, often uncomfortable, scared and sad. Still, it's enough to rethink the priorities of life and try to live the Hygge method to the best of ability, with healthy realism, but also with determination and maybe a little enthusiasm.

It is absolutely not true that nothing can be done against thoughts. We can to accept that it is our unconscious to direct the orchestra of our feelings, but we can take control of it and create the most suitable symphony for us to find happiness.

We just need to put any negative thoughts on a leash and leave room for positive ones: every moment of our experience is part of us and together with it we can grow, improve and discover ourselves. Imagine negativity as an angry beast: we are the sedative. Let's put it down and it will end up threatening us. We will have peace, the living space that will make us breathe serenely.

Each of us is a world in itself, and for this reason everyone is unique, important and indispensable. This can be confirmed when referring to tastes, passions and preferences. This is why it is right and healthy to have a job that is a perfect container for our serenity, lived with people who share our concerns and ideas. Nothing will overwhelm us.

Loving yourself is fundamental. Our mirror is an inescapable vehicle of self-criticism because on that side, reflections, we are there. We must appreciate ourselves, and a reflex is not enough: our body responds to our every impulse and we must never, and never, ever neglect it.

We observe a healthy diet, train, give our tissues energy and vitality. Sensations are like a flow: they can invest or overwhelm us, above all influence us. Meeting positive and lively people can give us serenity. We would therefore have no external problems to take on. The happiness of others can also become ours, because smiling is freedom. Our days will be more relaxed, and we deserve it.

We are indispensable to ourselves, simply. We avoid any emotional or material dependence. We need nothing more than our happiness, which only we can discover. Serenity, joy and smile are ours and we are masters of it.

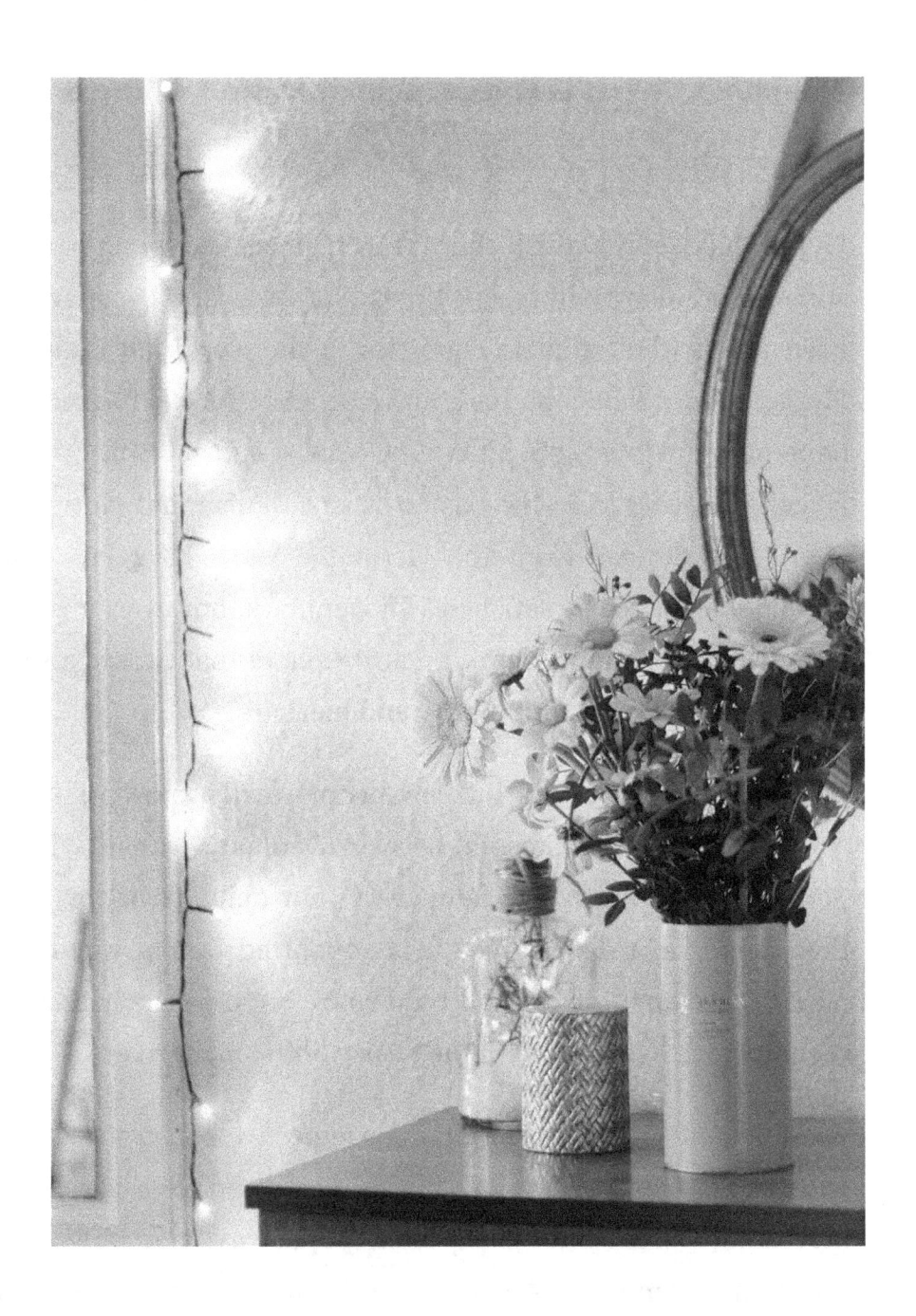

Chapter 1. What is Hygge, principles and where does it come from

Hygge is a deeply Danish concept, which has had an unexpected surge in popularity in recent times. For 40 years, Denmark has been one of the happiest countries in the world, all thanks to Hygge, a word that contains a universe and which is the secret of happiness for the inhabitants of this country. But, what is Hygge? Starting from the basics: it is a Danish and Norwegian word that derives from the Germanic word "hyggja" - that literally means "to be satisfied". In Denmark, however, it is used to indicate something more: an atmosphere that causes a sense of welcome, comfort, familiarity and pleasure.

Everyone talks about it, but few people really know what it is about: Hygge - this lifestyle born in Denmark, consists in the pursuit of happiness not temporary, but daily. A happy being that lasts over time because it is supported by the way of life itself. There are no fixed and rigid rules, but only the habits that seem to have been lost with the frenzy of the modern era.

Ever since it was included among the new words in the Oxford Dictionary two years ago, hygge has been experiencing a moment of great and unexpected popularity, not only in its homeland, Denmark. An incalculable number of articles have been written on this Danish word and why it is the key to

(Danish) happiness. It is no wonder that people are curious about it: on the other hand, the Danes are repeatedly at the top of the charts of the happiest countries in the world!

But what is hygge? The Oxford English Dictionary defines it as a form of intimacy that evokes a feeling of contentment and well-being, a fundamental concept in Danish culture. Many articles on hygge mention objects such as candles, hot chocolate and extra large sweaters, as well as being in the company of loved ones.

With the word Hygge we can define the ancient Danish tradition that makes every place and every moment special by creating a sense of intimacy and comfort. Hygge represents pleasure of a hot chocolate while it's cold outside, an afternoon on the sofa reading your favorite book or an intimate dinner with the people you love.

More specifically, the word Hygge is correlated with house, intimacy, and its atmosphere. For Danes, in fact, happiness revolves above all around their home, so they strive to make it welcoming and relaxing. Considering the very low and cold temperatures that occur, and the fact that days are short, the place where they live has a special value for the Danes. Those who follow the Hygge method find happiness in small things and do not "chastise" themselves, but give themselves small pleasures, pamper themselves and find time to dedicate themselves to those who love, cultivating interpersonal relationships. A lifestyle from which we should all take example.

Hygge is more than just a candle

Hygge is not just intimacy: it is a central aspect of Danish culture - and vocabulary -. In short, hygge is more important than a simple meeting with people you are fond of. Expressions like Hyggeligt a møde dig ("Nice to meet you") are used in everyday life. When children are played with their friends, it is said: "Hyg Jer!" (that means make yourself comfortable and relaxed). This is certainly not meant to suggest they light a candle or squeeze under a soft blanket. More generally, you want them to be well and have fun. You can even tell someone who plays video games!

The opposites of hygge and hyggelig are not uhygge and uhyggelig, as might be expected. Both words are present, but they mean "fear" and "scary". Furthermore, Hyggelig and uhyggelig are not mutually exclusive. For example, you can enjoy a hyggelig aften (intimate evening) with an uhyggelig film (scary film).

Language and cultural reality

It is not surprising that hygge has left its mark in the Danish language. Language is always a reflection of the people and communities who use it to communicate in everyday life. New words emerge when you need to describe new phenomena, words like "smartphone" or "Wi-Fi" are good examples. While others, such as "dowry", "telegram" or "steamboat", disappear from everyday use because they describe something that no longer plays a role in modern life.

In this sense, words and concepts deeply reflect the cultural history of a community. The Danish linguist Carsten Levisen centered his doctoral thesis on 20 words defined as key concepts for the language and culture of his country. There are words like hygge, of course, and then lykke (happiness), jantelov (Jante's law), and tryghed (security); all central linguistic concepts in the image in Danish culture.

An inaccurate meaning

It is worth noting that hygge is not the same for everyone: it is an individual feeling that cannot be defined clearly, and univocally, even among the Danes. The anthropologist Jeppe Linnet has been working on the concept of hygge for years and has realized that the precise meaning of the word depends on the social environment of reference. While for some, attending the local football club with friends has a high hygge factor, for others, it may instead be seen at the last show at the Copenhagen theater.

Much depends on the environments and social classes in which it is inserted. All the different hygge scenarios, however, have some things in common: a safe environment, people you are fond of and tasty food and drinks.

Is Hygge therefore untranslatable?

Not exactly. The word hygge can be satisfactorily translated into various other languages. And some aspects of the concept can also be found within other cultures. But the nuance of hygge that expresses security, equality and community is found only in the Danish language and reflects an important part of the image that the Danes have of themselves. Finally, to make everything more complicated, there is the fact that for each person there is a different and individual hygge.

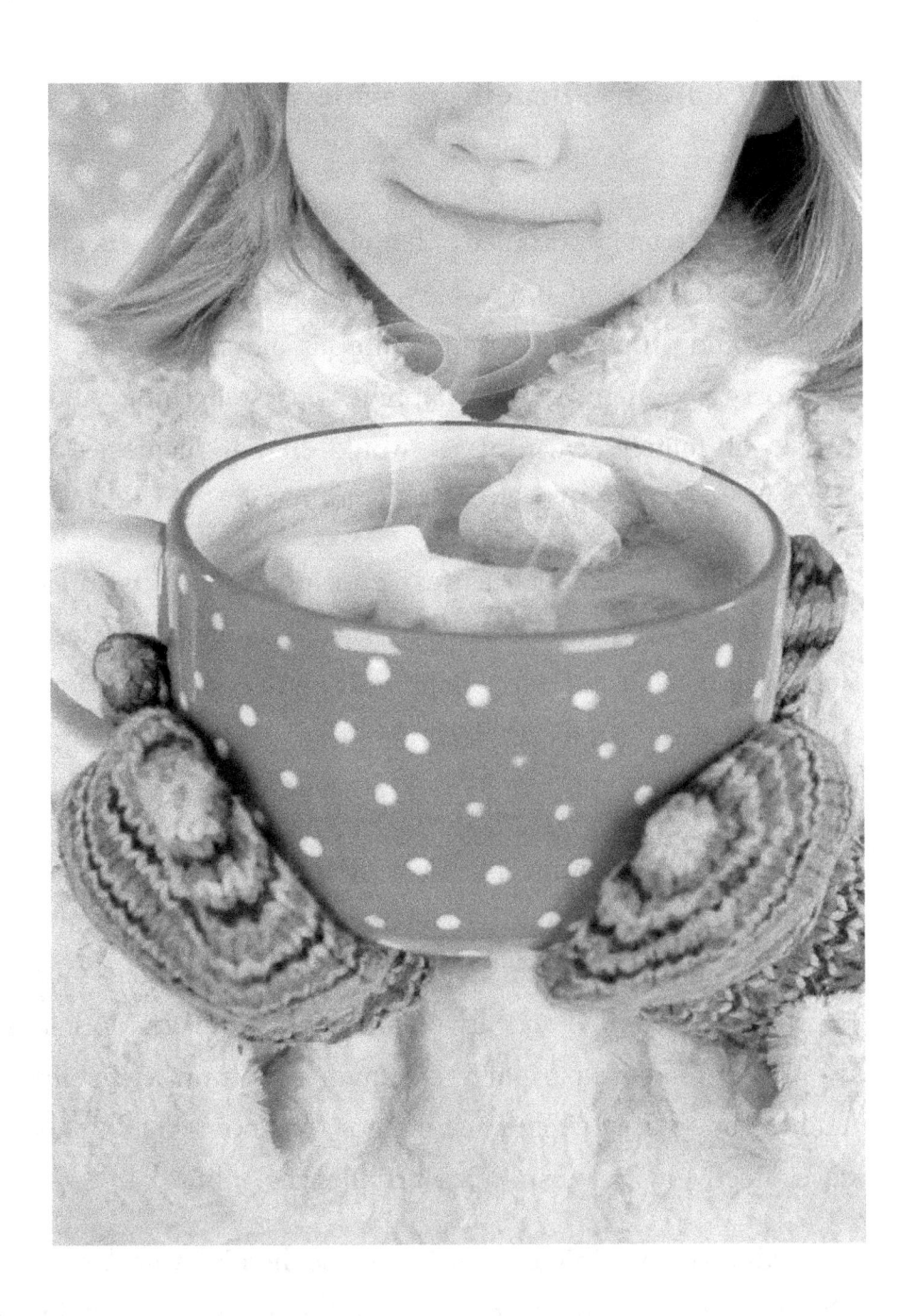

Chapter 2. Benefits of achieving happiness

What is the true importance of happiness? Happiness is not only linked to good mood, but also to health. Science now confirms it, while some people suggest there are far more important things to worry about, others see happiness as something vital, like what, ultimately, each of us would like to achieve in life. Happiness is more than a passing emotion.

Negative emotions, such as fear and anger, help us to escape from danger and defend ourselves from dangers. The positive emotions, such as pleasure, happiness and hope, help us connect with others and cope with negative situations that can happen in life.

Trying to live a happy life does not mean denying negative emotions or pretending to feel joy at all times. We all face adversity and it is quite natural to experience anger, sadness, frustration or other negative emotions. To think otherwise would be to deny part of the human condition. Being happy allows you to fully experience the positive moments, but also to face effectively the most difficult challenges of life.

According to Matthieu Ricard, the biochemist who became a Buddhist monk who is considered the happiest man in the world: "Happiness is not a pleasant feeling or a passing emotion, but an optimal state of being". According to the latest research, happiness not only makes us feel good in general, but also brings with it a series of benefits for health, relationships with others and performance at work.

Researches and economists from Warwick University, have shown that people who feel happy are more productive. Those ready to feel happy have shown themselves to be better able to perform the assigned work tasks. In the healthcare sector, doctors who are happy have been found to make faster and more accurate diagnoses. Schools that focus on children's social and emotional well-being also get better academic results. Happiness has also been related to better decision making and greater creativity.

Happiness also brings benefits for society as a whole. According to research based on the review of over 160 studies, there is clear and convincing evidence that happier people have better overall health and live longer than their less happy peers. They would also be less likely to get cold and have a heart attack or stroke.

Finally, happier people are more likely to make a positive contribution to society. They are more likely to volunteer and participate in public activities. They have greater respect for the law and offer more help to others. Success is the key to happiness, we usually hear ourselves say. Research seems to prove otherwise: happiness is the essential key to success. On the other hand, much or almost everything depends on us. The 90% of happiness is hidden in our mind: depending on how it processes the information it receives from the brain. So it can happen that people in tragic conditions are even happier than those who have an almost perfect life.

Even if the day started badly or something really went wrong, being in a bad mood will only allow you to quickly make matters worse. In fact, most of the time you become irascible, you get caught up in nervousness, negativity, you can't think clearly, it happens to you one after the other and with the people who are near you at home or at work it triggers a time when you bother each other: you become unbearable for them and vice versa. A vicious circle to lose.

But when you learn to be happy in spite of everything, the benefits you have are absolutely amazing. Obviously, I'm not going to tell you that you will magically stop having problems and that everything will run smoothly like new oil: those who live fortunately always face problems. What changes and improves is the way you will be able to approach what you live, they have also studied it scientifically.

Infact according to Doctor Barbara Fredrickson, a psychologist and researcher from the University of North Carolina, happiness increases visual attention and facilitates collection of information about what surrounds us. This, in daily life, personal and working, translates into a greater ability to solve problems; to find solutions; to come up with brilliant ideas.

The head is certainly a very delicate part of the human body, perhaps the most delicate as well as fascinating. It is the seat of the brain, of thought and of those endings that allow us to relate to the world around us. Precisely because of its centrality, receiving a massage in this area of the body is even more relaxing and beneficial, especially for those specific areas that can sometimes be painful due to the fatigue and stress that accumulate (typically the temples and the forehead).

We all love being well. It is one of the very few things that all human beings have in common, regardless of ethnicity, religion, political opinion. We like to feel good and positive emotions are simply good for us and characterize these states of well-being. You don't necessarily need a reason to fully enjoy it: simply ... we live them!

Experiencing emotions such as happiness, enthusiasm, joy, hope is fundamental for anyone who wishes to lead a healthy and happy life. To enjoy their benefits it is not necessary to try them at all times, even if these are the moments that lead us to think that, despite the effort, it is really worth it.

Being happy, from experience, helps you increase your emotional intelligence, that is, the ability to manage emotions, and also allows you to develop linguistic and interpersonal intelligence, because it allows you to better choose the words you say and also use with other people, who will feel "attracted" to you.

And that's another benefit: you're more attractive when you're happy! Happiness, in addition to being contagious, is seductive, because it gives more light to your expression, improves your posture, your pace and even your safety and self-esteem. Joy, trust, positivity, gratitude, enthusiasm, inner strength are just some of the feelings that brings you happiness and which in turn lead you to be happy.

Besides, did you know that happiness is better than a vaccine? It fortifies the immune system and therefore makes us stronger and more resistant to seasonal ailments (an experiment has been done in Pennsylvania confirms it scientifically, and also I, since I never take anything!). Here are 10 principles of a Hygge Style life. Maybe that's why Denmark is among the happiest countries in the world? Who knows ...

- *Hygge has at the center of its meaning the relationship between us and the outside.* A good atmosphere is important to activate the relaxation mechanism and a positive attitude towards life. Light is a fundamental element to create intimacy and serenity. Then, dim the lights, light one or more candles. Light and shadow reminds me very much of the Chinese Yin Yang principle, the interdependence of everything.
- *Hygge is the Danish definition of awareness: be here and be it now.* Turn off cell phones, television, radios. Stay in the moment without superstructures.
- *Hygge is also synonymous with our not to panic.* A life without drama is a life of peace. Rule number 2 can help us!
- *Hygge is pleasure of the mind, but also pleasure of body.* Treat yourself to something small and good every day. A chocolate, a cocoa bean, a coffee.
- *Hygge is social relationship.* Sharing of responsibility. Without the effort of imposing, everyone participates.
- *Hygge is gratitude.* The sun does not need to shine and everything should go smoothly. Even in difficult times, the heart can continue to believe that our life is special, for us and for others.
- *Hygge is harmony.* There is no jealousy, there is no abuse. Everyone is as good as he is, there is no need to

criticize or even brag.

- *Hygge is relaxation.* Balance, peace, fluidity. Contact with nature promotes well-being, as well as welcoming every season into your home. Don't run, stop and rest.
- *Hygge contains in its meaning the principle of solidarity.* We are not alone. We share our stories with others. We will learn and others will learn. Together.
- *Hygge means protection and refuge that comes from being together.* It is the meaning of our Tribe.

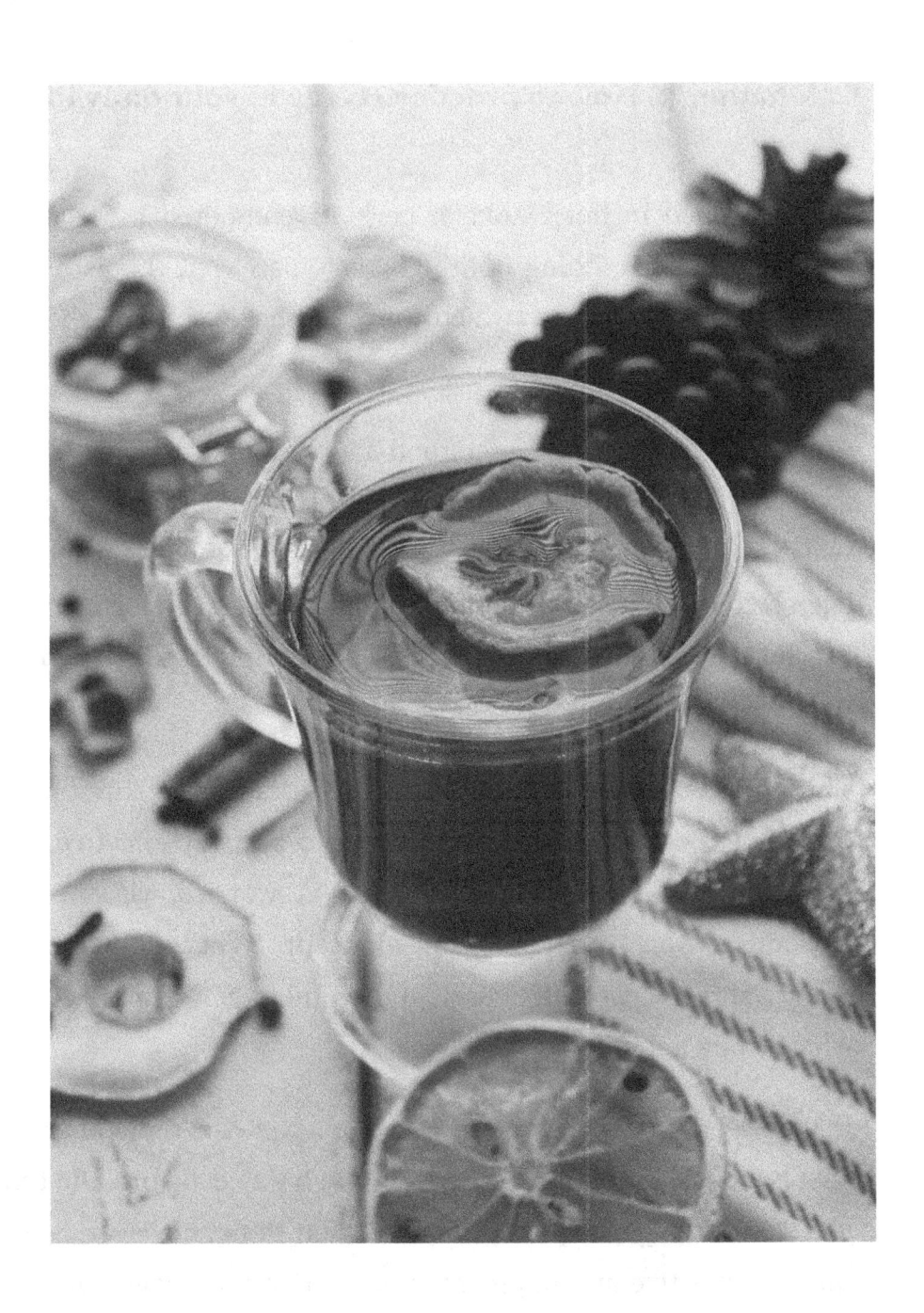

Chapter 3. How to practice Hygge in your daily life

Stay wrapped in hot blankets, perhaps pampered by a cup of steaming hot tea, doing nothing. Okay, sure, but this is only a small part of the hygge (which we read hugge). In fact, there is much more.

First of all, it must be understood as a moment to enter, alone, as a couple or with the whole family. In the period of time in which it is decided to do hygge (which can be half an hour or even a couple of hours) we do not talk about uncomfortable and thorny topics, that is, all those that could bring the discussion to light up.

Then, all the phones and devices (PC, TV, radio, etc.) are turned off. Why? Because in order for hygge to be truly effective, you have to leave everything else out. Via worries, via the last episode at work, via persistent whatsapp. When doing hygge, one must be focused on oneself and on the other, completely. So what to talk about?

If you decide to do hygge in company you can remember the past holidays, that fantastic dinner of two weeks before, the time you went to a special place: the important thing, however, is that they are positive and happy memories. If you do hygge on your own, a good idea is to practice deep breathing, but also to read good books. The goal is to regain possession of oneself and one's time, reaching a new serenity.

I have great affection and respect for the Nordic peoples. The simplicity of lifestyles, love for nature and a tendency towards the harmony of light makes them particularly fascinating in my eyes. There are no malicious comments or heavy negativity. Each helps the other so that not only one person does all work. Nobody takes pride in their successes, nobody attacks anyone, or competes with another. It is a balanced interaction based on the enjoyment of the moment, of food, of being together. In short, a refuge from the outside world. For some, the one just described may seem like a normal family reunion. For many, however, it is not.

These unwritten rules on the "hygge" factor are exactly what makes it so special. American anthropologists have been impressed by the "Hyggelig" interactions and the fact that nobody tries to take center stage. It is a moment when everyone takes off their mask and leaves the difficulties behind the door trying to appreciate the power of the presence of others.

There are mountains of research that support the importance of social ties for well-being. The feelings received and given to others are the meaning and purpose of life. Social bonds can increase longevity, reduce stress and even increase our immune system.

Researchers also found that Denmark's egalitarianism plays an important role. For example, a study by Robert Biswas Diener found that while wealthy Americans and Danes are equally happy, this is not the case for low-income Danes who are much happier than their American counterparts. Here are five "hygge" rules that you may want to apply to your life.

1. Be yourself. Let your guard down. Don't try to prove what you are not.

2. Forget disputes. You prefer lighthearted and balanced discussions. Enjoy food and company.

3. Think you are a member of the team. Collaborate and work with family or group members. Help them prepare dinner.

4. Look at the hygge factor as a refuge from the outside world. A place where everyone can relax and open their hearts without judging and being judged, no matter what is going on in your life. For better or for worse, this place is sacred and problems can be left out.

5. Remember that Hygge factor is limited in time. Hygge can be difficult for a non-Dane. Take center stage, brag or complain, be too negative and try to be present without arguing? These are

very difficult behaviors to implement, but the reward could be huge. It's an incredible feeling to share these hassle-free moments with the people you like most.

Hygge is simply this... A deep sense of well-being, warmth and intimacy that we experience in certain moments. The warmer a place and the serene atmosphere, the greater the chance of being happy. Being alone, at home, with a good book and a herbal tea is particularly hyggelige, but in company it is easier to be. Being with other people, three or four, not large groups, sipping a glass of wine.

Eating sweets, conversing serenely, without having to appear or prevail over others, these are the people you need to surround yourself with to be happy. Hygge is also this, sharing. For example, cooking together, walking in the open air in company, dining at home on cold winter evenings. Doing activities with friends or family, organizing themed evenings, the heart of Hygge is found within the home, in our refuge.

Objects help to create a hyggelige atmosphere, the more "lived", dated, the more Hygge is. From a warm scarf that wraps you, to a wool sweater that you use for Sundays with your family, to an old pair of Christmas socks. Here all this leaves a sense of harmony and serenity. Because old objects are perhaps associated with a memory, with the memory of a happy moment from the past. And remembering a peaceful situation always leaves a nice sense of tranquility. As well as the furniture, from a particular lamp to a blanket that is dusted off every winter. The key word is: tradition.

The best seasons for Hygge are undoubtedly autumn and winter, when the days begin to get shorter and the temperature drops. Sitting in front of the window as the sun sets and admiring the light reflecting off the orange leaves that have fallen from the trees makes it all special.

Even walking in the woods collecting chestnuts can help you be happy. Moving away from technology, cell phones and the internet, it is essential to be able to notice what is really important: small things.

The most Hygge moment of the year, however, is Christmas, which even has its own term: Julehygge! This term is used to describe the Christmas atmosphere. The Danes in fact love Christmas and organize everything according to the hygge, they talk about it continuously and the countdown to December 25th is a real party.

Family and friends, Christmas decorations, from elves to Santa Clauses, candles and hearty food are fundamental parts for a truly hyggelige Christmas, without these ingredients Julehygge would not exist.

So let's summarize: winter, candles, fireplace, warm cover and blankets, pajamas, book, more candles. Herbal tea, cinnamon cakes, the people we love. These are the basic parts of Hygge. Wherever you live you can reproduce the Danish lifestyle with these simple tricks!

And ok, maybe we won't become the happiest country in the world, but at least we will bring in this way some serenity and happiness into our lives. Because we all need a little warmth, love and to pamper ourselves in order to feel good.

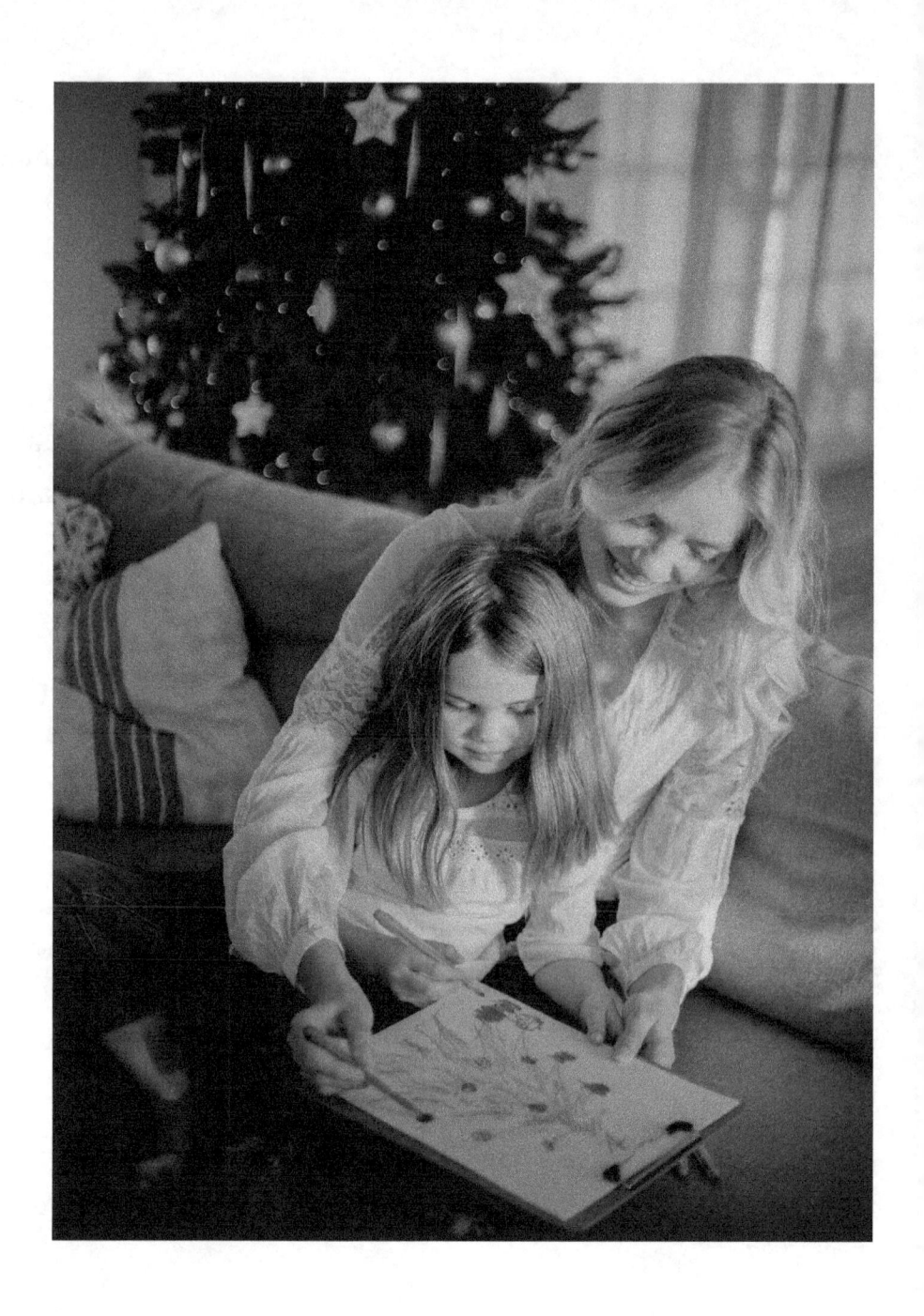

Chapter 4. Hygge style at home: how to turn your home into a "happy refuge"

Happiness is a warm and fragrant corner, within the home walls. Hygge is the Scandinavian way of living happily. Here's how to apply it to your home to make it warm, welcoming and comfortable. The key to living better and longer is scientifically proven: a warm and welcoming home that induces us to slow down and relax, puts us at ease and makes us happy because we are satisfied simply by what we have.

The Happy Research Institute of Copenhagen, which studies everything can make us happier, from the correct lifestyle to nutrition, and which identifies in the "domestic heat" one of the three key factors for living in a qualitative way, together with social security and well-being of body and soul. Feeling good about yourself, feeling "at home", protected and safe, happy with what we have has its definition - the Danish word "hygge" (pronounced hue-gah): that feeling of warmth and protection that we can only feel , do not describe, and which is intimately associated with the house, the family nucleus, at the beginning and end of the day.

Therefore, recipe for happiness exists, and very little is needed to implement it and experience its benefits in person. A cup of coffee in the morning, a lunch in the living room, a book read on the sofa near the crackling fire, a hot bath at the end of the day: hygge is all this and the feeling of well-being to be shared in harmony with relatives, family and friends in obviously suitable environments. And considering that this trend is no longer a Danish prerogative, why not take advantage of the intimacy and warmth of the house during the winter to make it more welcoming and comfortable all year round?

Well thought-out spaces and banished disorder. A first step in embracing the hygge philosophy is certainly to be aware of the spaces by letting them talk about you and take care of the house. Consider what you have and what you can add and change to make it more welcoming, instill this awareness in all members of your family, including children, and try to invest in intelligent solutions to contain the disorder and keep what you don't use frequently. Remember that the hygge space is also quiet and harmonious, also and especially in the colors.

Living in a hygge way means making the home a meeting place, for a stress-free exchange of opinions, opinions and ideas, always in a relaxed way, meeting friends and family in a peaceful oasis setting. And specifically the Hyggekrog is a part of the house where you can spend time in a hyggeligt way. There are also ten things that make the house more hyggeligt:

- Place in the house, usually in the living room, where you can sit between the cushions with a blanket;
- Fireplace;
- Candles;
- Wooden objects;
- Nature;
- Books;
- Ceramic objects;
- Coatings of different workmanship;
- Vintage furniture;
- Pillows and blankets.

Hygge Light

Lighting in home is essential. To create a warm and welcoming hygge atmosphere, it must be dosed and - above all - as natural as possible. If your home has dark corners, revive it with the warmth of a candle light, especially in the evening, for example by taking the habit of putting one or more on the family dinner table.

A personal corner

Fundamental to the psychological well-being of the human being is the possibility of having a personal place that functions as a welcoming refuge when living one's own home. As children we experience it and ask for it without filters: a room all to ourselves, where we can give life to our world. As adults it can be more difficult to defend one's own space but it is necessary to do so. Create a corner of the house that is only yours: an armchair with your favorite plaid on it, a table with your magazines and books, your teapot. Imagine yourself there when you're out and about to go home.

The ideal temperature

There is nothing more welcoming than a warm house in winter. A good boiler can be a perfect investment (choose one with extended warranty, to ensure maximum peace of mind). Always use it with awareness and moderation: you must manage the internal temperature so that it is warmer and more enveloping in winter, but never dry. Improve the air quality in your home by using essential oils and humidifiers to spread a good revitalizing and comforting aroma in all rooms.

A mug of tea and a book

Happiness today is increasingly "off-line". Being able to afford the luxury of disconnecting the phone and not looking at the email, even for just a couple of hours, really regenerates. Make sure that your pantry is stocked with fine tea and invest in a nice teapot. Allow yourself the luxury of going out to buy (in person, not via the internet) a novel that you are passionate about. Spend two hours, every weekend, to your happiness at home with your favorite book and hot tea. Top up your batteries wonderfully. Equally effective is the favorite DVD version + chocolate cake!

Design and order

Everything in its place and a place for everything: an orderly and clean home environment makes you happier. Spend a day cleaning up your home environment with the space-clearing technique. Throwing away (or putting in the attic) is often the best cure for the stress of disorder that crowds our lives. Then reward yourself by buying a design object you have long desired: lamp, small table, desk furniture or that electric kettle that you have never purchased.

A quality bed (even aesthetic)

The quality of sleep reflects on our life and our daily happiness, but having a good mattress is not enough. What is your bed like? Look at it and give it a frank score: it must entice you to spend a comfortable night and a few mornings in total laziness. If not, invest in a new pair of sheets (crumpled linen sheets that don't iron are very practical) and a good number of decorative pillows. A plaid to put on in contrasting color helps to make everything even more comfortable.

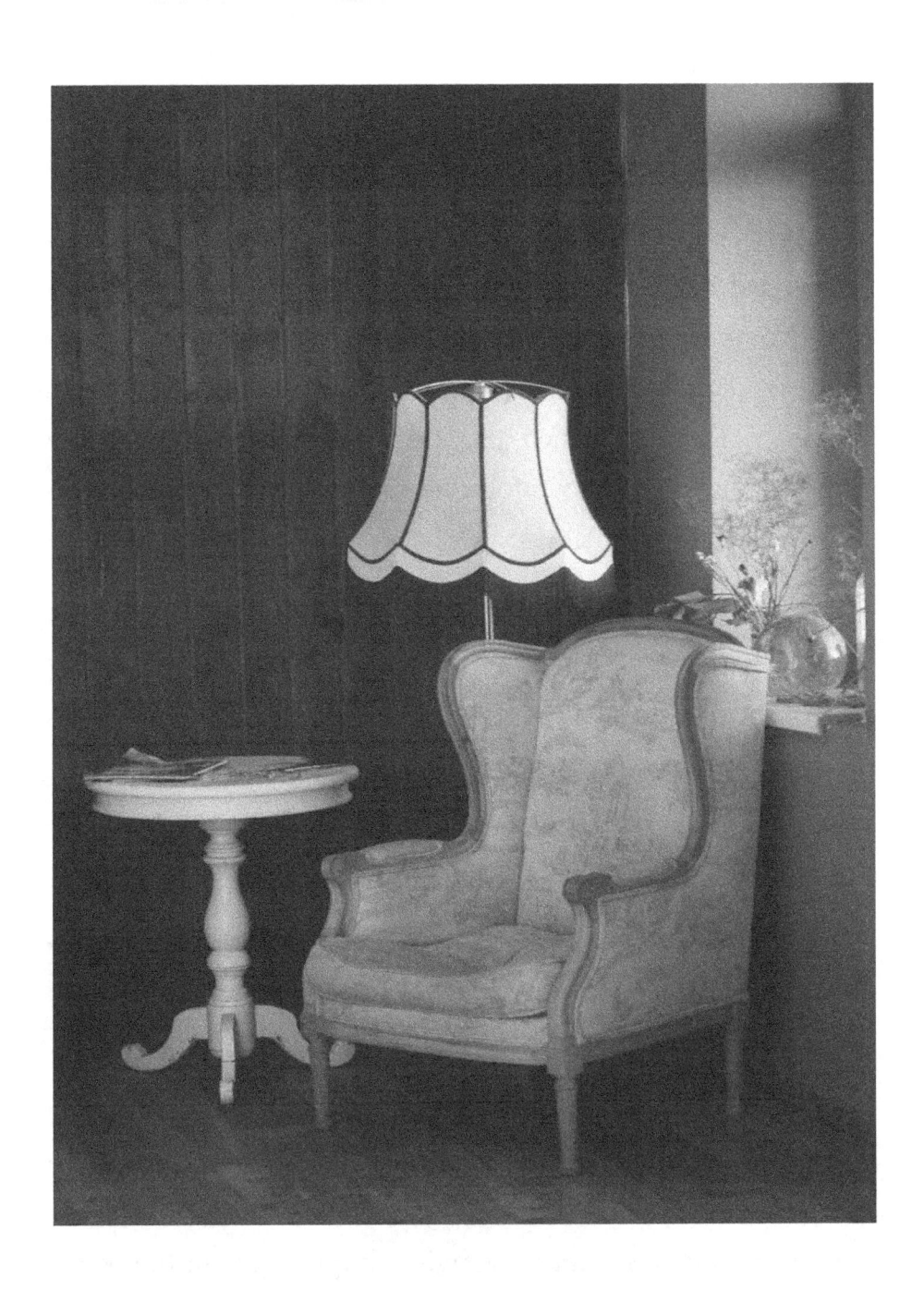

Barefoot (at home)

One of the most hygge sensations that can be experienced is a gesture that we make daily, but sometimes without being fully aware of it: taking off our shoes. Make your home offer a bare environment to your bare feet, especially when you wake up. A soft carpet to rest your feet on when you get out of bed, a warm wooden floor on which you can stand barefoot in the living room. And a pair of comfortable socks with which to run around the house, without shoes, always.

Living well in a cozy home, tailor-made for us, is not something we can do, but we must do. Hygge is to live happily by enjoying the pleasure of the little things that we often take for granted. It is an art that can be applied to our entire life and therefore also to our home. Yes, because it is not so difficult to furnish a Hygge-style home. No huge expenses are needed, just a few small tricks.

Hygge style bedroom

In bedroom, the choice of furniture is focused on the search for the bare minimum, without unnecessary frills. Enjoying life with a few simple things means having ample space in the bedroom, so go ahead for small wooden wardrobes, needing a few essential clothes while a carpet on the edges of bed will make getting into the bed warm. A simple painting with themed tints is the only decorative element of a single-color wall. Alternatively, the use of wood allows to cover the wall with a warm and enveloping effect. A bedside table on which to place small personal items and a small lampshade lamp, is the functional element of a poor room. For lighting the bedroom, low-impact solutions such as floor lamps and lanterns where to place small candles are ideal for making the atmosphere relaxing and even more romantic.

Hygge style lounge

Focusing on creating a relaxing environment in the living room is imperative for those who choose this style. It is in fact the meeting and relaxation place par excellence, and it must be made as soft and comfortable as possible with sofas, cushions, seats, to facilitate people in being at ease.

A large soft and thick pile rug, on which to lie down, pampering yourself with large cushions, useful as seats and to rest your neck and back while, in the winter seasons, woolen blankets and plaids allow you to stay warm if there is no fireplace in the living room, traditional element in Danish houses. There is no shortage of sofas and armchairs, especially in the models with chaise longues that allow you to relax, relax to rest or read a good book in front of the fireplace.

If you love design in particular, armchairs with curved and sweet lines, with wooden structure are perfect for a corner of the living room or a classic rocking chair, on which to rock for short and deserved relaxation.

Hygge style kitchen and dining room

These rooms are also dedicated to moments of sharing, furnishings privilege the essentiality and the space to be dedicated to guests. A large wooden table, with benches made comfortable by large cushions, facilitates entertainment while preparing something hot, a dessert or an improvised aperitif.

To enjoy moments of conviviality with friends, you don't need pomp and immoderate luxury: simplicity best combines with natural materials such as wood, therefore, recycling old chairs is definitely a great way to create DIY furniture in hygge style. Ideal a kitchen overlooking living room with an open space that makes conviviality easier while preparing recipes.

There must be an adequate number of chairs, with a series of folding, so you can comfortably store them in a closet or in a little used corner of the environment when not needed.

Hygge style bathroom

The place to relax and dedicate yourself to body care. The only room in the apartment where you are used to being alone, furnishing and equipping the bathroom in a soft and relaxing way is not complicated in itself. Compared to the more practical shower, the tub is ideal, being able to immerse yourself for a long time without any hurry. Small accessories such as a mirror on the wall and a ladder for storing towels and bathrobes will be more than enough for the relaxation area.

A few simple precautions for the rest, starting with the colors chosen to paint the walls which, in the wake of the Nordic and Scandinavian style, favors for kept and clear colors, primarily white. Simplicity is also combined with the choice of materials, with wood making the figure of the protagonist.

A light stool, preferably crafted and left in its natural color, is a practical support for small personal items while in the tub. To create the right atmosphere, scented essences released into the environment help to relax the nerves and relax while from a small radio, soft and fusion music will be the ideal side dish.

Hygge-style balcony

Spending free time outdoors is the best way to meet friends. For the arrival of summer, it can be sufficient to create a relaxation corner on the balcony or terrace of your home. And even if the small size may create some doubts, the basic philosophy of the hygge style is to relax with little: a sofa, if necessary also a model of the inflatable ones, a folding table or a shelf that can be attached to railing, make the space suitable to entertainment even on a balcony. A ceramic pot with green plants, a lantern and a carpet will be the right and ideal complement.

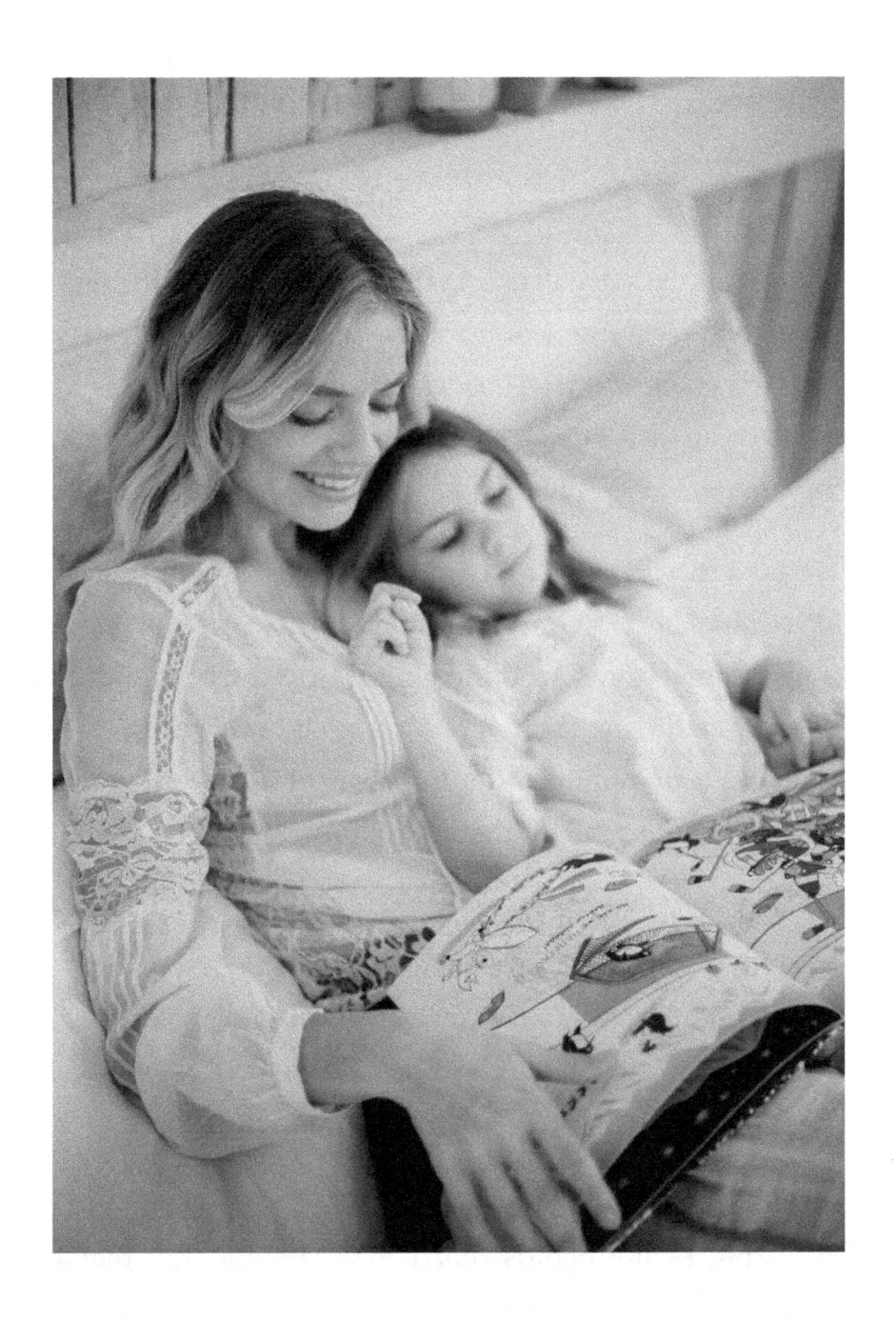

Chapter 5. The Danish method of living happily applied at work

First of all, let's say that bringing Hygge to all situations in our life is really easy and to do so we simply have to translate the rules (very pleasant!) That we already apply at home at other times of the day. Above all, at work. To make our work and our professional place super Hygge, just a few gestures are enough.

We take care of our desk making it pleasant and welcoming, a little more fun and less minimal (but without necessarily transforming it into something messy). We bring, for example, a cup from home, without buying it on purpose: it will unconsciously remind us of the comfort of our intimate spaces (and it will be useful for the next point!).

Hygge is also very much about friendships and relationships, to be cultivated with love: that's why we should always try to bond with our colleagues (with whom, if we think about it, we really spend a lot of time in our lives!): We take it as a habit the coffee breaks together (with our snuggling cup) and let's treat ourselves every now and then to an aperitif with them.

We bring family photos that make us smile and that fill our hearts, arranging them on the desk in nice frames (not simply gluing them on the wall in a sad way, unless we choose stylish washi-tape, like these or these).

Let's not forget, however, also indoor plants, because one of the rules of Hygge is that which involves bringing nature inside! To maintain that sense of warmth not only emotional but also physical that is typical of Hygge, we keep a nice wool blanket under the desk: sometimes colleagues prefer cool but we are cold? It will no longer be a problem, and you too will appreciate the opportunity to crouch in the wool.

Hygge is family, and therefore even when we are at work it is better not to lose sight of her. We appreciate the time spent there, trying to feel good and make the days pleasant, productive and complete, but then let's not forget about our house: we avoid too many overtime and, like the Danes, we always leave work at the set times, not late.

In this way we will all have time to enjoy our home and family, the stress will be reduced and we will also be more productive, as well as in peace. There are those who manage to work with a background music and those who cannot. In any case, if you love low music surrounds you, try to create a soft and relaxing, warm and acoustic playlist (using online services we can now create all types in a very simple way; for example we use either Spotify or Amazon Music Unlimited).

Whenever possible, we go out for lunch taking schiscetta outdoors (always with colleagues!): Even if we don't miss the green plants on the desk, spending time on a lawn is always a relaxing pleasure. Finally, let's not skimp on compliments: being an Hygge guy means being welcoming and above all, literally, means thinking or feeling satisfied.

Even a small compliment sometimes works wonders: it creates a virtuous circle of kindness, instills self-esteem, and there is nothing more pleasant (and productive) than a workplace on which everyone feels appreciated and valued. So, let's summarize some essential tips for living Hygge outside the home, at work and in the office.

1) Take care of the desk. Make it tidy but less minimal than the classic office desk. Occupy it with a scented candle or an ambient fragrance that recalls the atmosphere in the house, maybe you use the same one. How about a cup? A nice one, the kind that you use for breakfast and that make you feel once again in a more welcoming environment than the working one. Hygge teaches that it's always a good thing to bring nature "indoors", so why not choose a small plant for your desk? Opt for a cactus, it will bring color, freshness and good mood.

2) Live the lunch break. Do not eat at your desk, forget the days when, to optimize time, you stayed in the office, in front of your

PC, during your lunch break. Lunch must be a moment of relaxation, tranquility and leisure to carve out during the work day: eat in the open air or in a place under the office. If there is a park near your workplace, go in the middle of nature to enjoy lunch in solitude or in company, the only rule: do not talk about work.

3) The digital detox. If your office work involves long-term contact with computers, social networks and the web in general, a break from digital is needed, the so-called detox. So take advantage of lunch to unplug the phone and enjoy only your well-deserved break.

4) The blanket. One of the things I learned with Hygge is that the feeling of well-being on cold winter days is given by the "cold outside and warm inside". Even in the office it is possible to feel the sense of emotional and physical warmth of the Hygge: take a woolen blanket and keep it close at hand so as to pamper yourself on the coldest days.

5) Human relationships. Hygge is family, friends, human relationships. Building relationships with work colleagues is just as important as everything else. Try not to talk only and exclusively about work, rather share with your colleagues small daily joys of your life. Be welcoming with them and do not spare smiles and compliments, especially towards more difficult

colleagues. You also appreciate the work of others, your behavior will be an added value for you and for others.

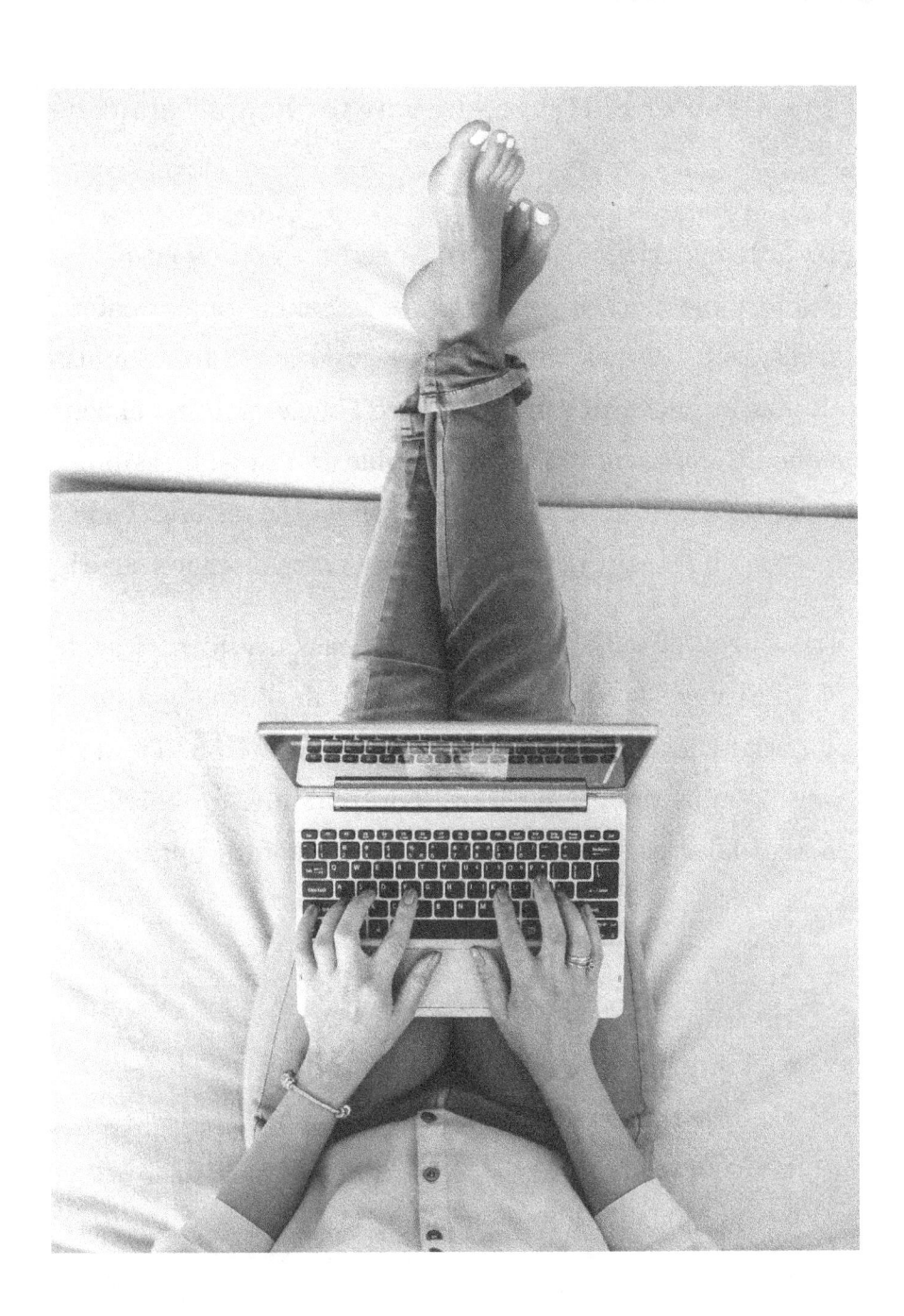

Chapter 6. Hygge, the way to "happy" clothing

To fully experience Hygge you need to be dressed in the most comfortable clothes you have: loose pants, long sweaters, wool socks, soft clothes, dressing gown and t-shirt. Sophisticated clothes are not worn to experience Hygge, nothing expensive or signed is necessary, Hygge is humble and slow: it is simplicity. It is watching from the window while the strong wind blows outside and covering yourself with a grandmother's shawl.

The hygge style? But of course a casual and easy style! The Nordic style is minimalist, simple in lines, comfortable in materials, mainly natural like wool and cotton. The feeling of well-being is preferred rather than pursuing formal elegance. It is a casual style. The must have elements of the hygge:

- Scarves, stoles and wool shawls;
- knitted sweaters;
- wide trousers like pajamas or pajamas;
- wool socks;
- handmade objects - handmade-.

Hygge and me

Hygge for me is not a discovery ever tried, on the contrary, it corresponds very much to my lifestyle, the discovery was instead to find a name that identifies a situation, a feeling and that helps me to fully and consciously live emotions and special moments .

Beauty in the book is finding a series of recipes to recreate it, to look for it, to bring it into everyday life and thus be truly more grateful and happier. And after all what are we looking for if not the happiness and love of living in sharing with loved ones?

The Danish women, with their enveloping and soft outfits, have become true style icons to be inspired by for the cold season. Here's what to copy from their wardrobes for a living fashion.

Hygge. A word difficult to pronounce, almost impossible to translate ... but all to live. What is it about? It is not something that can be touched or seen. It is something that, quite simply, can be felt. It is, in fact, a feeling, a warm and safe feeling, a state of profound well-being.

It is the basis of the Danish method and is based on the harmony of a community, on happiness cultivated at all times, on the ability to savor the little things in life.

In Denmark, this particular attitude to well-being and happiness is sought after and translated into many aspects of everyday life, which thus become tools for feeling good and living in full hygge style. The wardrobe is obviously no exception: it is precisely from this philosophy that Danish women have developed their own way of experiencing fashion, thus becoming true style icons, especially in the more casual fashion dedicated to every day. Here are 4 things to copy absolutely from their outfits, to bring a little hygge spirit and a touch of authentic Danish style in your wardrobe.

Soft hugs ... made of wool

Warmth and comfort typical of the Hygge philosophy also enter the wardrobes in the form of soft weaves. Here, therefore, that wool becomes the most present fabric in the wardrobe of Danish women and takes on different shapes, comes in different weights, gives us different processes.

It simply becomes the indispensable cozy touch to pamper yourself from head to toe. Sweaters and pullovers therefore, but not only: also dresses, joggers and coats. The softest total looks ever come from Northern Europe, to warm up even the coldest winters with a comfy-chic sparkle.

The Danish palette

The palette to bet on for a perfect Danish style? It is composed of 50 shades of black, there is no doubt! Black and all shades of gray are in fact at the base of Danish women's wardrobes, which tend to show off total black or total gray looks with a lot of ease in the most disparate situations. Their secret? Playing with textures and overlapping elements, for a personal and never boring or flat effect.

If you are not a lover of the very classic black, however, do not worry: the alternative obviously exists and is composed of natural and neutral colors, such as light beige or white. And the color? It is not totally banned from the wardrobe, but should be dosed with extreme caution and used mainly in spots, for example on small accessories such as hats or scarves.

Volume games

Overlaps, are very popular with Danish women. Practical, full of charm and personality require the use of amiably oversized garments, truly ideal for bringing a pinch of Copenhagen to any wardrobe. Knitted maxi dresses, loose pullovers and oversize parkas are in fact authentic cornerstones for a self-respecting hygge wardrobe. Have fun playing with the contrasts of volume therefore, remembering however to always balance very large garments with others that are very dry. A few examples? An oversize cardigan in thick wool superimposed on super skinny jeans or a maxi dress in cashmere worn with low socks and bikers, easy to replicate and carry.

Comfy accessories

The accessories most chosen by Danish women fully reflect the practical and cozy spirit of the rest of the wardrobe, there is no doubt. The real must haves? Scarves and caps. In soft wool, braided or ribbed, they enter right into the play of volumes and material contrasts, completing the outfits and becoming absolutely essential details, perfect for warming up and pampering the coldest winter days.

And on your feet? The shoes par excellence are quick, fast, very comfortable. In a word: sneakers. Choose them to wear with jeans and joggers, but also to complete the more girly looks, with protagonists in maxi dresses in knit or skirt ... they will become ideal companions for your days, as well as perfect touches of style to play down any outfit with a pinch of good humor. Get the look!

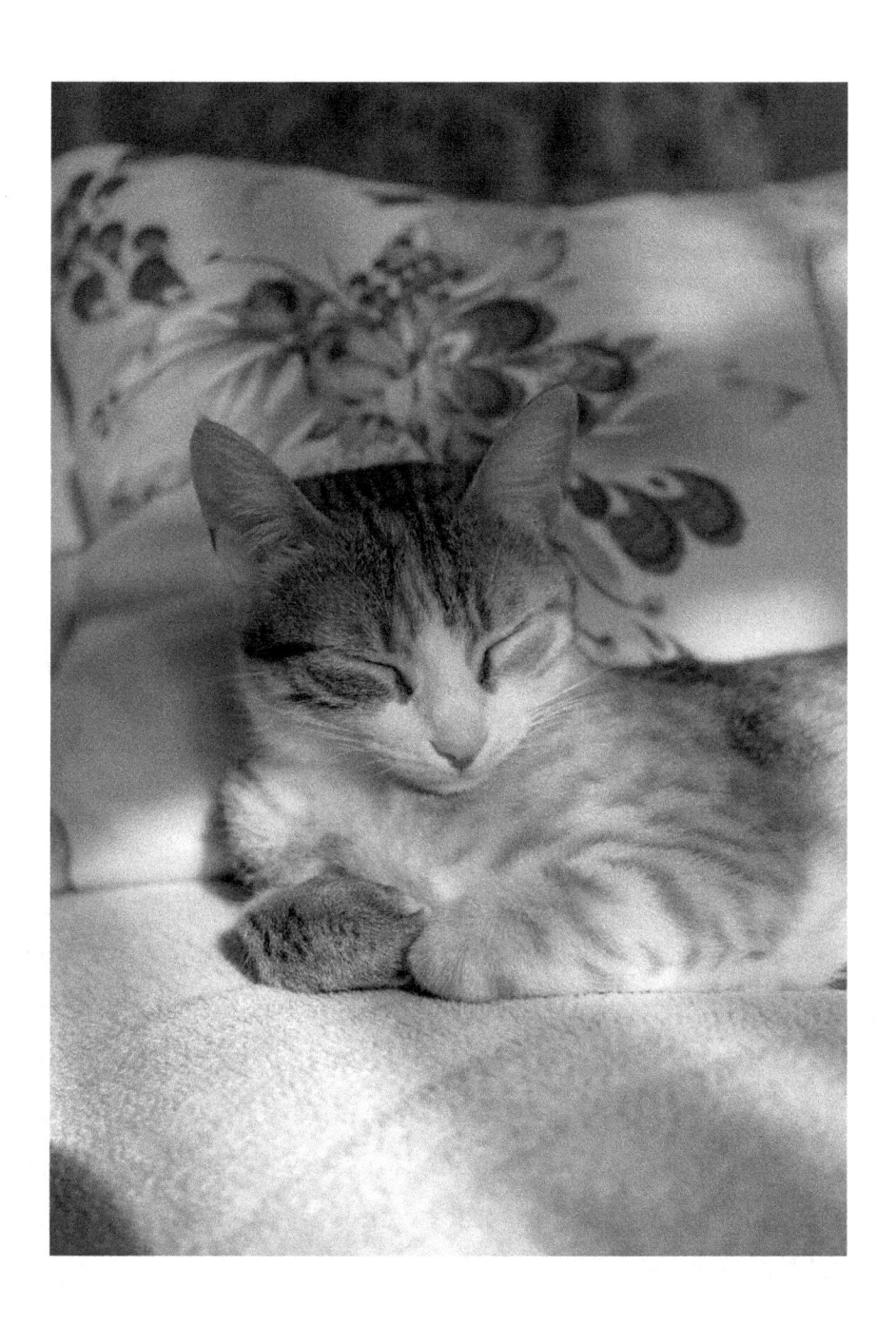

Chapter 7. Hygge inspirations for cooking

It is now fashionable to talk about Hygge lifestyle, this untranslatable Danish term means to live life without stress, enjoying the little things, giving yourself moments of happiness even through simple gestures, everyday like choosing a relaxing furniture, filling the flower house, spend time in the middle of nature. Needless to say, this lifestyle also involves culinary field, the act of cooking and sharing a meal are moments to live in harmony, looking for pleasure even in what may seem repetitive gestures, it is part of the Hygge thought for example to put aside the excuse of - I don't know how to cook, I don't have time - to take care of yourself.

Sign up for a cooking class within your reach, not only will you learn new notions and recipes but it will also be a means of meeting new people, socializing, or creating a sort of rotating kitchen with friends, colleagues, relatives, useful for not stressing and living moments of conviviality. Be open to new flavors, cultures, taste unknown dishes, be curious to experiment with new combinations, try to taste an ingredient that does not excite you, enjoy calmly the moment you sit at the table.

Recipes in full Hygge style, we speak of Danish dishes but obviously the ideas are endless, the smorrebrod, it is bread buttered with avocado, eggs, salmon, shrimp, vegetables, sprouts, cheese, usually it is made up at the moment, a fun moment in which the imagination is stimulated in creating one's own we call it improperly sandwich.

The cinnamon swivels, the Danes are used to indulging in a sweet treat once a day, swivels but also chocolate, marzipan, cream, butter cream, a small greedy moment to fully enjoy.

Another important role among Hygge dishes, soups, with fish, vegetables, spices, legumes, rice, cereals, hot dishes that heat up and can be prepared in many variations; meatballs, usually accompanied by potatoes and presented with gravy, beef, venison, game.

The glogg, a hot drink typical of the Scandinavian countries, made with wine, spices, sometimes almonds, recalls our mulled wine. No matter what the recipe is, to lead a Hygge lifestyle you just have to prepare it with taste, pleasure, perhaps in company, totally savoring the flavor and comfort it gives you.

In fact, what makes hygge magical is sharing, being together, feeling surrounded by affection as when you are at the table with dear friends. What are the foods that according to the Danes are more reassuring and can transmit this feeling of warmth? We also discover 10 recipes that can help us feel better, especially when the temperatures drop drastically, it is bad weather and the days are getting shorter.

- Hot chocolate: what could be more reassuring and pleasant than holding a cup of hot chocolate sunk in your armchair at home? Maybe in the same place where grandfather used to read fairy tale books to you when you were little. All of this is hygge and can be recreated in minutes. For a perfect hot chocolate mix the cocoa powder with the milk. Separately melt a few pieces of dark chocolate. Bring the milk to a boil and add the melted chocolate.

- Fish soup: it is a classic of Scandinavian cuisine, a warm pleasure that pampers the stomach and spirit. It is not by chance that soup recipes are widespread in all cultures. Based on vegetables, legumes, rice, cereal, spices: so there are many possible variations. Denmark, surrounded on three sides by the sea, could only make a very common raw material such as fish the star of this recipe. To this are added carrots, celery, leek and garlic. Finally, the cream that guarantees creaminess and makes a dish of poor origin more substantial.

- Pea soup (gule ærter): it is a Danish recipe that has more than 200 years of history. In these centuries it has brought comfort and warmth to thousands and thousands of people, starting from the countryside up to the exclusive restaurants of the capital. In fact, many variations are developing from the traditional dish, from the simplest to the most refined and sophisticated ones. The base remains of yellow peas. Traditionally, to add more flavor and substance to the whole, pork is added.

- Meatballs: another dish present in different traditions, ready to wrap our taste buds in a soft embrace. The most famous Scandinavian Scandinavian meatballs are of Swedish origin but it doesn't matter, all of this is hygge. Usually minced pork, beef or game is used and everything is presented with a thick roast sauce, an element that certainly makes our recipe more succulent. Don't forget the side dish of boiled potatoes, another symbol of Scandinavian cuisine.

- Cinnamon rolls: they are similar to American cinnamon rolls. What is the difference? That the Danish recipe is not filled with dried fruit. What makes these soft sweet loaves special is the intense aroma and flavor of cinnamon. After all, isn't it the aroma that reminds us more of Christmas, the moment of the year where you feel (or should feel) the warmth of your loved ones more? Start the day with a cinnamon bun and a cup of filtered coffee or tea. Your awakening will have a completely different flavor!

- Rye bread (rugbrød): the smell of freshly baked bread is certainly one of the most reassuring and good in the world. In Denmark this intoxicating aroma takes the form of loaf bread. It is dark, prepared with rye flour. The surface (sometimes even the crumb) is sprinkled with sunflower seeds. You can eat it simply with a layer of salted butter spread on it or make it the base of the smørrebrød, the Scandinavian open sandwich. When it is a few days old, use it to prepare a porridge.

- Smørrebrød: according to many, this simple slice of stuffed bread is able to give off positive vibrations ... it is certainly a simple and rewarding way to have lunch. It is a dish that lends itself to a thousand variations and that can be easily shared with friends and family. Smoked or marinated salmon, hard-boiled eggs and shrimps, pâté, cheese, smoked mackerel, herring, avocado ... are all ingredients that can make your lunch very hygge. Are you ready to try?

- Gratin dishes: fish (usually cod), cabbage or potatoes au gratin would make anyone feel at home and in any place. Here is the essence of hygge! The ingredients, before being cooked and browned in the oven, are sautéed in a pan with butter and then covered with a soft cream cheese or béchamel sauce. Very popular is also the Bernese sauce, of French origin, prepared with yolk, butter and white wine.

- Roasted pork (flæskesteg): this type of meat has always been one of the most popular ingredients in Denmark, along with fish, potatoes and cabbage. In particular, roast pork is the typical dish that masters Danish tables for Christmas. The tasty and crunchy crust makes it really inviting! As flavorings, pepper and bay leaves are simply used and everything is served with cabbage and potatoes.

- Glögg: we started by talking about the hygge drink par excellence, sweet hot chocolate. We cannot end with another warm, highly comforting liquid pleasure. Have you ever heard of glögg? It is a Scandinavian spiced wine reminiscent of mulled wine. Some, however, add, in addition to spices, raisins and almond flakes. Then there are those who appreciate a drop of rum or cherry liqueur. No matter the recipe, the important thing is that it is a simple moment of pleasure to be shared in joy.

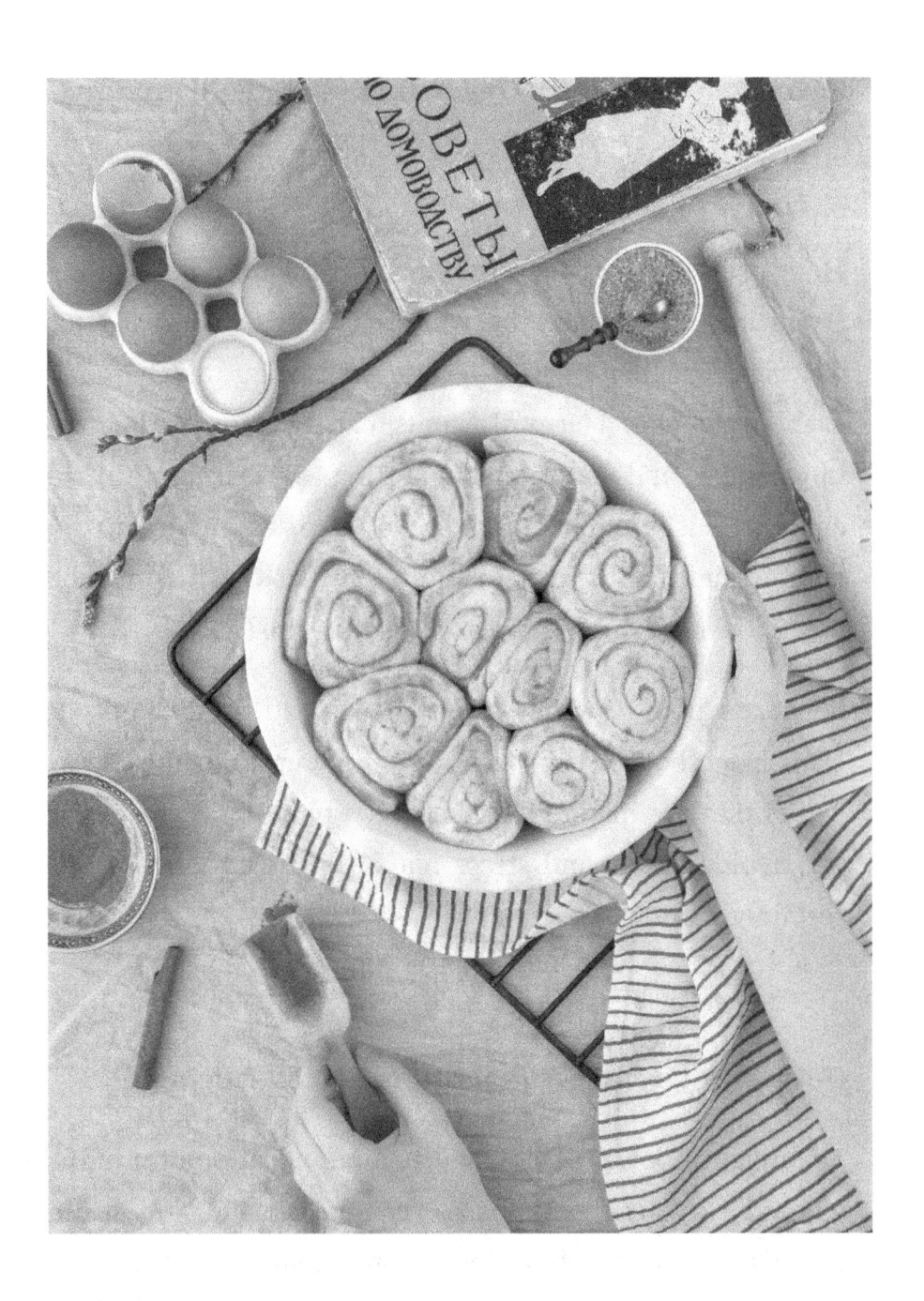

Chapter 8. Healthy Hygge habits to avoid anxiety and stress

Here are some practical hygge-style tips to avoid anxiety and stress and better face the winter. Lifestyle can really make a difference on the level of health, well-being and happiness of each individual. Harmful habits can encourage the onset of imbalances and emotional suffering. If learning to manage emotions is fundamental, it is also essential to include empowering habits in your daily life that can help to obtain a greater level of satisfaction and self-esteem.

So here's how to be happier and less stressed thanks to the Danish method of happiness. Try to start from these 5 simple habits that are inspired by the hygge philosophy, they will help you avoid anxiety and stress making your days (and your life) certainly more pleasant.

Get rid of stress with emotional decluttering

The magical power of tidying up, an application of mindfulness method to your living spaces, can be a valid anti-stress aid. Discover all the benefits of conscious decluttering and how to do it in your life. Starting from home is easier and will help you take the first steps to get to a real inner work. To reduce anxiety and stress, tidying the house is in fact a real cure-both for the mind and soul. Cleaning outside (and inside) of you will help you feel greater inner freedom and lightness and live the present with more serenity.

The anti-stress power of tidying

Cleanliness and order will help you make the environment in which you live more comfortable and your home will be free from energy stagnation. The same goes for working environment, where a free mind is even more creative, relaxed and productive.

Dedicate yourself to the usual reorganization, avoid accumulating things that risk blocking the energies of the home and your unconscious. Get rid of old objects you do not use (especially if related to past emotions that could upset you) and keep only what is really essential with you. The art of letting go can also be learned in this way, putting this principle into practice in your home will also help you do it within yourself.

Remove anxiety and stress by creating the right atmosphere in your home

To create harmony in the environment in which you live, you can use light to heat the spaces of the house and adapt them to their functions. For example, if you place your work environment in the most illuminated and exposed to sunlight to promote energy and concentration, it is better to illuminate the areas dedicated to relaxation and rest with soft lights.

Your home is your mirror, make sure to make the environment you live intimate and warm. Adjusting the brightness of your home helps you not to accumulate tiredness, avoid anxiety and stress (and keep winter depression away). The nervous system is affected by light and with this little trick your sleep and your mood will improve considerably.

The salt lamps help you clean the air and the energies of the house and give a pleasant and regenerating atmosphere, light them before sunrise and sunset to relax and add candles to encourage meditation. In this way you will make the environment more welcoming and the atmosphere more intimate, even relationships will be influenced in a positive way.

At the table seek pleasure (to nourish the mind and body)

Eating healthy does not mean depriving yourself of taste, on the contrary you can enjoy tasty dishes focusing on healthy and various spices and condiments, typical of the Mediterranean diet. Warm and enveloping food like spicy cereal and legume soups will help nourish your mind, warm your body and spirit.

Indulge in comfort food you love, perhaps in a light version, to avoid anxiety, fear and stress leading to attacks of emotional hunger. Experiment with new recipes to add more taste and health to your kitchen. You can get used to enjoying hot tea and herbal teas (perhaps in company) to carve out moments of relaxation. Follow hygge tips for your relationships.

Immerse yourself in nature and listen to its subliminal messages

We are part of Wild Nature and the seasons influence our psyche and our emotions. Each season invites our unconscious to make a profound change. If autumn invites us to let go, to close the cycles and to gratefully reap the fruits of what we have sown, winter suggests that we slow down the pace and recover our inner energies.

Seasonal fruit and vegetables, thanks to precious vitamins and trace elements, will help you strengthen health and vitality starting from autumn. During the winter, adding these foods to your diet will help protect your body and mood by removing anxiety and stress due to the change of season. But how to deal with this busy life?

Get used to taking nature walks (in a park if you live in the city) and get inspired. Natural landscapes help to meditate, stimulate reflection and introspection. Being silent will encourage deep listening, will help you regenerate your energies. Many scientific studies suggest that being in nature has beneficial effects (a help at no cost to avoid anxiety and manage stress).

In fact, nature helps to reduce stress and, negative thoughts and to balance emotions even for the most impulsive characters. Also known to science are its restorative effects on cognitive skills that are more compromised during the winter.

Against anxiety and stress insert your sacred hour in each day

Try to dedicate at least an hour of the day to what makes you feel good. Even better if you manage to get up early in the morning and immediately create a space for yourself and your inner well-being before commitments and duties take over. You can enter in this sacred space:

- a few minutes of meditation and emotional healing practices to free the mind and nourish the spirit;
- a short session of yoga or exercise to connect the mind and body;
- reading a good book that gives you the right inspiration to start your day in the best way.

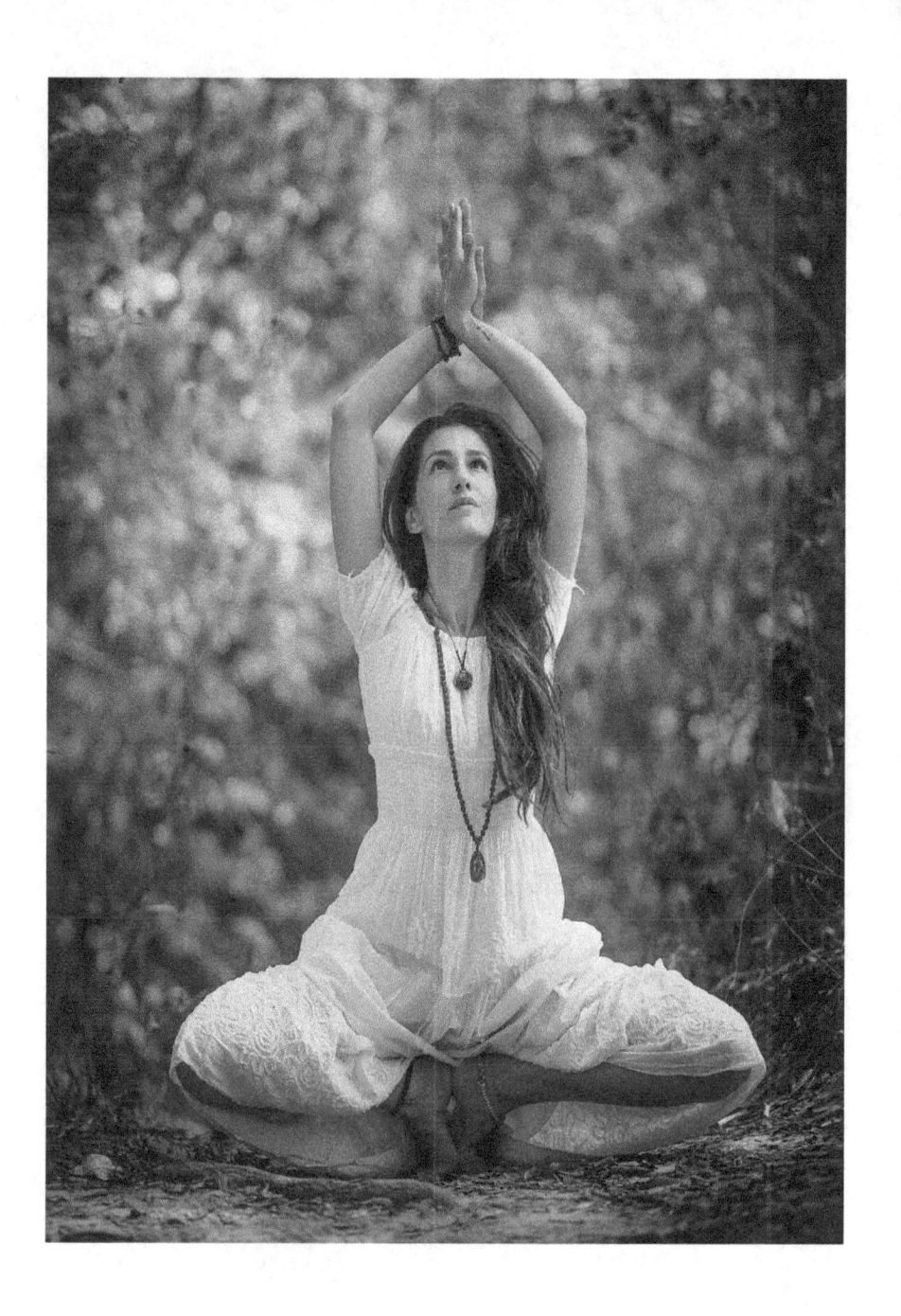

Spend time on your passions

Find the space in your day to do what you really love so you will avoid anxiety and stress in your life. It is precisely when you lead a life too full of duties that you risk incurring emotional suffering that can result in psychosomatic symptoms or panic attacks (this is in modern times one of the most common diseases in the western world).

Summing up

These are the 5 empowering habits to remove anxiety and stress inspired by the hygge method:

- Free yourself from stress with emotional decluttering: you will learn to let go of negative emotions as well;
- Create a relaxing atmosphere in your home: to make the place you live intimate and welcoming;
- At the table, she seeks pleasure (to nourish the mind and body): anxiety and stress are also won with the right nutrition;
- Immerse yourself in Pure Nature (listen to its subliminal messages): let yourself be regenerated by the healing powers of green spaces;
- Enter your sacred hour in every day: dedicate yourself

every day to your inner growth without ever neglecting what you love and make you feel good.

I hope these tips will help you avoid anxiety, stress and sadness that are more frequent in winter. I hope they can inspire your days to add more well-being and happiness to your life.

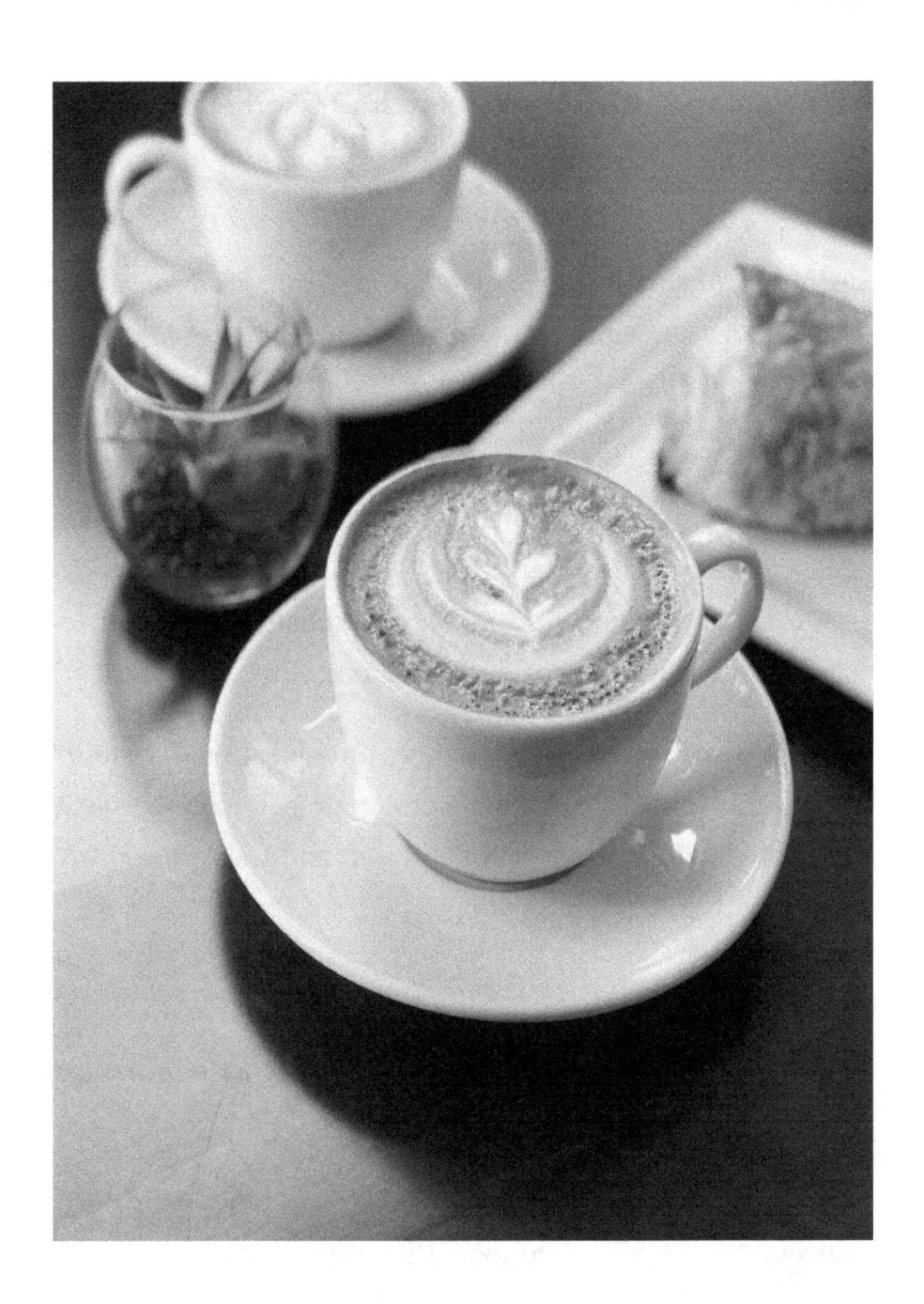

Chapter 9. The Danish method to educate children about happiness

Before going into the Danish method, let's start with a fundamental premise. The dream of all mothers is to see their child happy, but:

- Can you educate to serenity?
- Can you be taught to be people who are formed in the name of happiness?
- Is there an educational and behavioral system to deal with life and phases of childhood with this positivity?

The Danish method is not simply an educational system to be applied at school, but a behavioral approach to be permeated in the daily and social fabric of children and their parents. A path to live satisfied and raise happy children.

Educating children about happiness in school and in life

What makes our children happy children? I want to start from an episode of my childhood that occurred within the school walls to reflect on suggestions that derive from the Danish method. In elementary school I had a math teacher who made me hate the subject, in the sense that I was convinced I didn't have the neurons to understand it! The checks were conducted by making us put real barricades around desks, so as not to copy. It was only allowed to go down the corridor after the class assignment.

All this acted on the sense of competition (with the "let's see who finishes first" effect) and certainly did not feed support and mutual aid. I was terrified of that approach and for five years I never went to corridor. The discomfort generated was never expressed to the teacher, my anxiety, the sense of inadequacy and the profound insecurity in feeling "inferior" to my companions.

Listening to the empathic soul was completely missing.

Here, this pedagogical method is diametrically opposite to the Danish one, summarized with the acronym *PARENT* to underline how decisive the role and peaceful and relaxed attitude of parents is. School is just one of many environments where educational system can be applied, which in reality embraces all phases of everyday life, therefore also family, friends and society. School teaching given by knowledge of the subjects is not the only relevant element and is accompanied by the development of other specific skills in the child.

Live happily with the game

At this point you are wondering what the secret of happiness is. The key is free play. Through this activity the child is trained, vents, develops, learns to manage the various tests and to face his fears. Playing is one of the principles of inspiration of the Danish method PARENT which translates into:

- Play
- Authenticity
- Reframing
- Empathy
- No ultimatum
- Togetherness

How much do we influence our children with the choices we make?

As a parent I wonder about my attitude and choices I make for my son. I've been wondering since the days of pregnancy. I wonder how much my reactions can influence, inhibit, hinder or encourage the growth of child. The message that I "take home" from Jessica Joelle Alexander's book is contained in four macro areas: I find them useful tips that are good for mom, dad and baby.

- trust
- empathy
- sincerity
- courage

Trust. Key concept that is reached through self-esteem. The latter, as already mentioned, is determined by free play, by the possibility of experimenting, trying, testing. Children breathe our anxiety, so we try to remove what scares us, the dangers are often our problems and not theirs. Doing so, we avoid putting negative feelings on children. Undoubtedly useful to assign children to do tasks such as tidying a room or preparing the table, this encourages them to bring respect for the place where they are. One point that really made me think is the "award ceremony". What attitudes should be rewarded? Instead of praising them for the vows they take, it is more constructive to recognize the value of kindness, the collaboration they show and gratify these gestures.

Empathy. How to create a good climate where children can experiment? Thanks to empathy we lay the foundations for a healthy environment, where no one is judged, but only seen, taken into consideration, listened to and involved in order to naturally nurture a sense of belonging. I take my cue from my bad, traumatic experience as a primary school girl to emphasize how important it can be to learn to read yourself and others, listen to your feelings and feelings. Again thanks to an empathic fabric in which adults raise children, emotional honesty is transmitted, not the pursuit of perfection.

Sincerity. This aspect intervenes incisively on the climate of serenity. It means letting children know the truth about everything. Even on topics often thought to be inconvenient such as death or sex. This pushes to become more aware, helps to grow resilient and serene and in some way more in tune with your person. Here the ability of adults to relate to their children without taboos takes care of communication. Discover the tips for raising a child who speaks with parents.

Courage. In the Danish method, the courage to make mistakes is trained without being afraid of judgment. The attitude to try, risk, experiment and get back into play is always cultivated. By doing so, we allow ourselves the opportunity to learn from our mistakes and grow strong. The nature of this constructive approach is undoubtedly exciting and leads to success in terms of quality of the path followed and not as a synonym of perfection. The proposed lifestyle leads to the growth of happy children, feeds their involvement in the community by feeling an active part and consequently facilitating the progressive reduction of bullying.

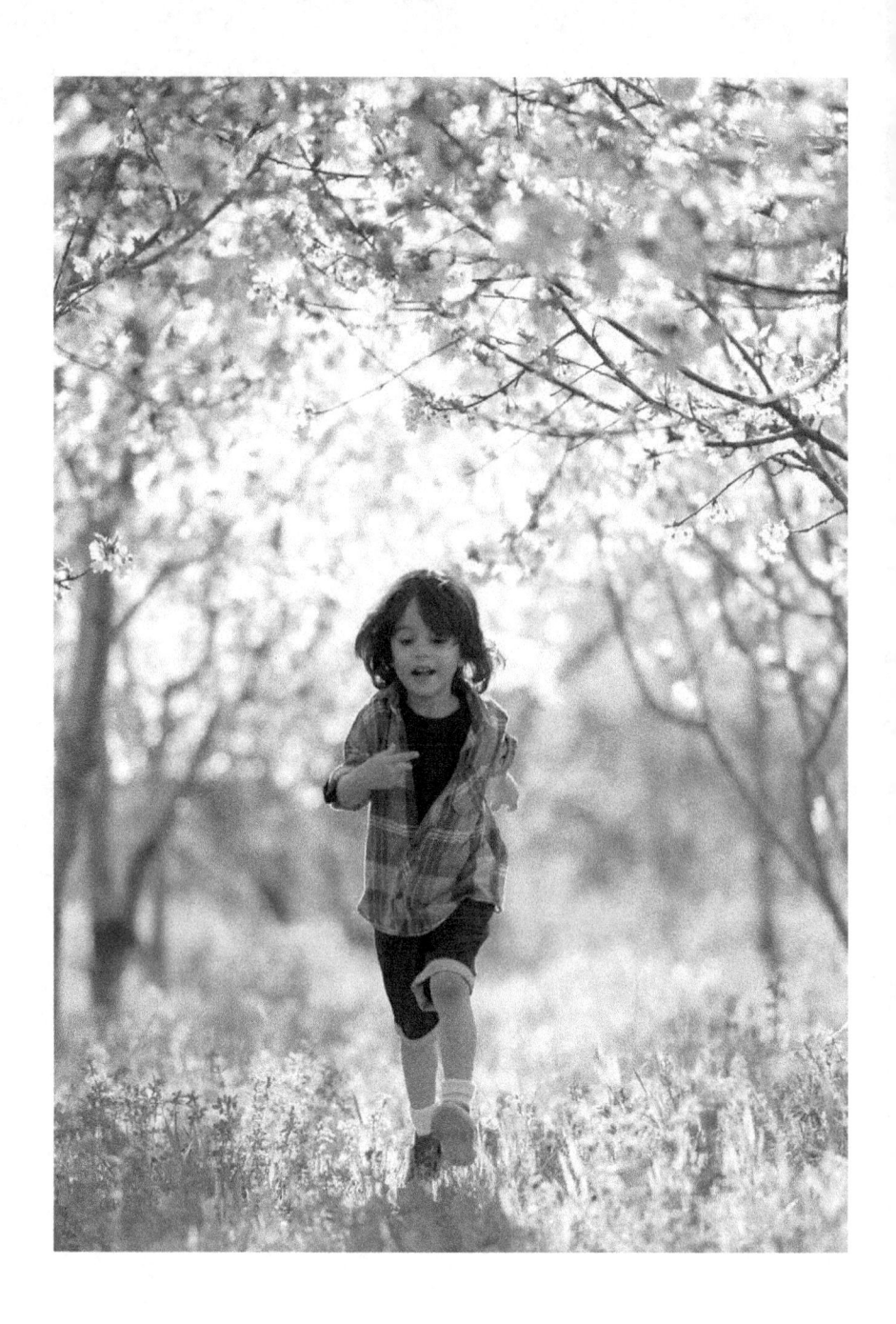

Chapter 10. Positive emotions and our wellness

Before going into the analysis of positive feelings and emotions, let's make sure we all have the same wavelength as regards this issue. It is not simply a matter of "happy feelings" to be pursued to experience momentary pleasure; moreover, like their negative counterparts, they also play a key role in our daily lives.

There are many ways to define the term "emotion"; these are the main ones:

- Emotions are a state or feeling that cannot be evoked at will.

- Emotions are attitudes or responses to an objective situation or fact. (Zemach, 2001).

Most current researchers prefer the second definition and consider emotions as the result of an event provoked by an action. The implications between preferring one meaning over the other are interesting, however, for the purposes of understanding the nature and role of positive emotions in psychology, it is not necessary to opt for a choice between proposed definitions: they are their effects are of most interest.

Limiting ourselves to positive emotions only, there are two common definitions, very similar to those proposed. They are, in fact, defined as "short-term multi-component response tendencies" (Fredrickson, 2001), roughly aligning with the second possibility, and "as intense and pleasant mental experiences" (Cabanac, 2002), adhering to the first. Or, positive emotions serve us "to broaden our awareness and strengthen our inner resources". This is the crux of Barbara Fredrickson's revolutionary "Broad and build" theory of positive emotions. Read on to learn more.

Whatever definition you like, the relevant information to know is:

(a) what emotions it is,

(b) what is their purpose,

(c) how we can best experience them, in quality or quantity, and

(d) the effects they have on us.

The list of positive emotions experienced is almost infinite; not all the words listed can refer to the emotions properly understood by scholars, however, these are those most used by people to describe their state, and this allows us to have an excellent starting point for understanding how they are commonly experienced.

- Joy - a sense of euphoria, happiness and sometimes hilarity, often experienced as a sudden excess due to a positive event.
- Gratitude - being grateful for something specific or simply all-encompassing, often with humility and reverence.
- Serenity - calm and peaceful acceptance of oneself.
- Interest - curiosity for something that catches the eye.
- Hope - optimism and expectation for a better future.
- Pride - self-approval and pleasure for an achievement, skill or personal attribute.
- Fun - carefree pleasure, often accompanied by smiles and laughter.
- Inspiration - sense of contentment, relief and motivation towards something that has been witnessed.
- Wonder - emotion evoked by seeing something great, capable of unleashing a sense of overwhelming appreciation.
- Motivation - a feeling felt when you observe someone engaged in actions of kindness, generosity or inner goodness, and that pushes you to want to perform a similar action.
- Altruism - usually indicated as an act of generosity towards others, but it can also describe the feeling felt in helping others.

- Satisfaction - pleasure obtained from realizing something or satisfying a need.
- Relief - happiness experienced when an uncertain situation evolves for the better, and a negative result is avoided.
- Affection - emotional attachment to someone (even to pets), accompanied by sympathy and a sense of pleasure felt in their company.
- Cheerfulness - feeling of radiance, of visible happiness, as if everything is going well.
- Surprise - joy felt when in receiving unexpected happiness or when a situation evolves better than expected.
- Trust - strong sense of self-esteem; it can be specific to a situation or have a more universal meaning.
- Admiration - approval, respect and appreciation for someone or something.
- Enthusiasm - sense of excitement accompanied by motivation and commitment.
- Desire - less intense form of enthusiasm; feeling of readiness and excitement about something.
- Euphoria - intense sense of joy or happiness, often experienced when something extremely positive and exciting happens.
- Contentment - peaceful, comforting and discreet

happiness and well-being.
- Entertainment - pleasure for what is happening around us, especially in situations such as recreational or group activities.
- Optimism - positive emotion of hope that encourages us to look to a better future in which to believe that things will turn out for the better.
- Happiness - pleasure and satisfaction for the natural evolution of events; sense of general enthusiasm for life.
- Love - perhaps the strongest of positive emotions, love is a feeling of deep and lasting affection for someone, combined with the desire to put others' needs before their own; it can refer to a single individual, a group of people, or even to all humanity.

This list contains a good part of the positive emotions experienced, but it is certainly not an exhaustive list - surely more can be added! Now that we have an idea of the type of emotions we are talking about, we can move on to another important question: what is the purpose?

Why do we need positive emotions? What benefits can they bring?

In addition to making us feel good, positive emotions are also a fundamental part of the puzzle of happiness. Based solely on temporary and hedonistic pleasure, we will probably not achieve lasting happiness; positive emotions can instead be the basis for those fleeting moments that make life worth living. For example, the joy of saying "I do" to others, the love that overwhelms holding your child in your arms for the first time, or the immense satisfaction that you feel in reaching a professional goal.

Although it seems that positive emotions have no other purpose than to make us "feel good", they actually play some very important roles. What is acquired and developed through the experience of positive emotions has proven to produce many benefits in different areas of life. In the vast field of physical and psychological health, positive emotions can have fantastic effects. We all love being well. It is one of the very few things that all human beings have in common, regardless of ethnicity, religion, political opinion. We like to feel good and positive emotions are simply good for us and characterize these states of well-being. You don't necessarily need a reason to fully enjoy it: simply ... we live them!

Experiencing emotions like happiness, enthusiasm, joy, hope is fundamental for anyone who wants to lead a healthy and happy life. To enjoy their benefits it is not necessary to try them at all times, even if these are the moments that lead us to think that, despite the effort, it is really worth it.

The effects of these emotions are in stark contrast to those of negative emotions, typically experienced in dangerous situations (e.g. fear, terror, anxiety), which usually have the effect of restricting our attention and limiting our myriad of possibilities to those , few emotions, suitable for survival. In such situations, automatic responses are vital; however, if you are not life threatening, such a narrow perspective in terms of options is not necessary.

It is in this case that positive emotions are more advantageous: instead of limiting our abilities, they expand them to allow creative thinking and action. Instead of narrowing our attention to a few answers, they broaden our awareness to accommodate a much wider range of possibilities to choose from. This expansion of our horizons allows us to learn and acquire lasting knowledge and skills. They can be physical, emotional, psychological, social and even mental resources, but, regardless of the type of resource acquired, they will be durable.

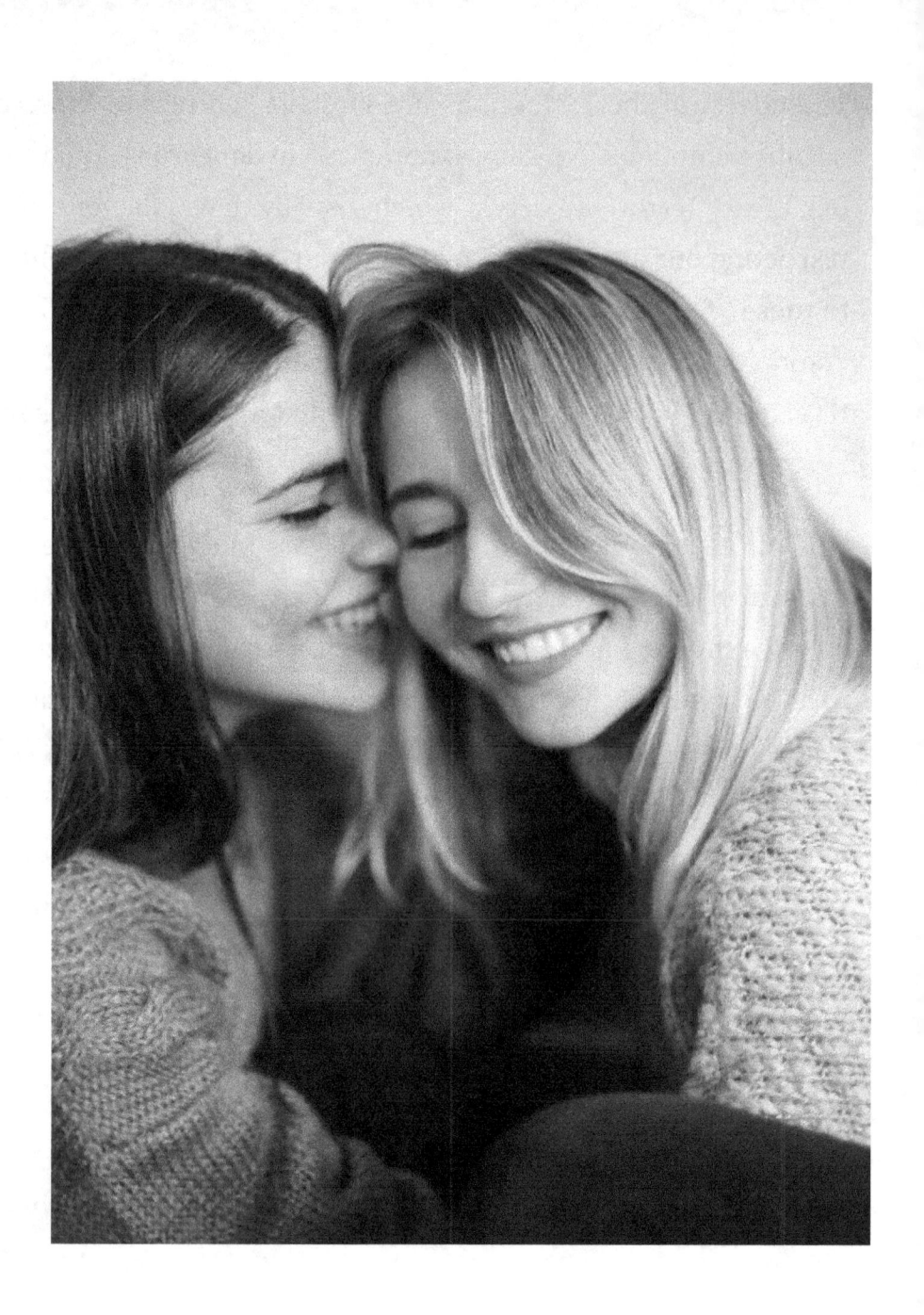

The benefits for health of positive emotions

Among the many health benefits there is a reduction of stress and a boost to general well-being. Positive emotions can actually act as a barrier to stressful events, allowing you to deal with them more effectively and preserve mental health (Tugade, Fredrickson, & Barrett, 2004). In addition, the researchers confirmed in 2006 that experiencing positive emotions helps modulate the reaction to stress and allows you to recover more quickly from its negative effects (Ong, Bergeman, Bisconti, & Wallace), enhancing your resilience capacity.

Positive emotions can also protect against sinusitis! Students who were causally assigned the task of writing about intense and positive experiences for three days (20 minutes a day) developed significantly fewer symptoms of the disease than students who wrote texts on neutral subjects (Burton & King, 2004). Experiencing positive emotions can also encourage individuals to make healthier decisions, indirectly helping to improve their health. Following some of health benefits:

- Happiness derived from an increase in behavior oriented towards the search for variety and to receive.
- The satisfaction generated by behavior focused on risk prevention.

- Positive emotions can also improve health by providing a barrier against depressive symptoms (Dolphin, Steinhardt, & Cance, 2015).
- Furthermore, being aware and taking the time to savor positive emotions can provide additional protection against the symptoms of depression, while increasing psychological well-being and life satisfaction (Kiken, Lundberg, & Fredrickson, 2017).
- Another health benefit is the ability to strengthen your heart

Kok and colleagues (2013) found a connection between a healthy heart rate and the experience of positive social emotions. Similarly, a meta-analysis of several studies has verified that well-being is significantly related to good cardiovascular functioning, general health and longevity in general (Howell, Kern, & Lyubomirsky, 2007).

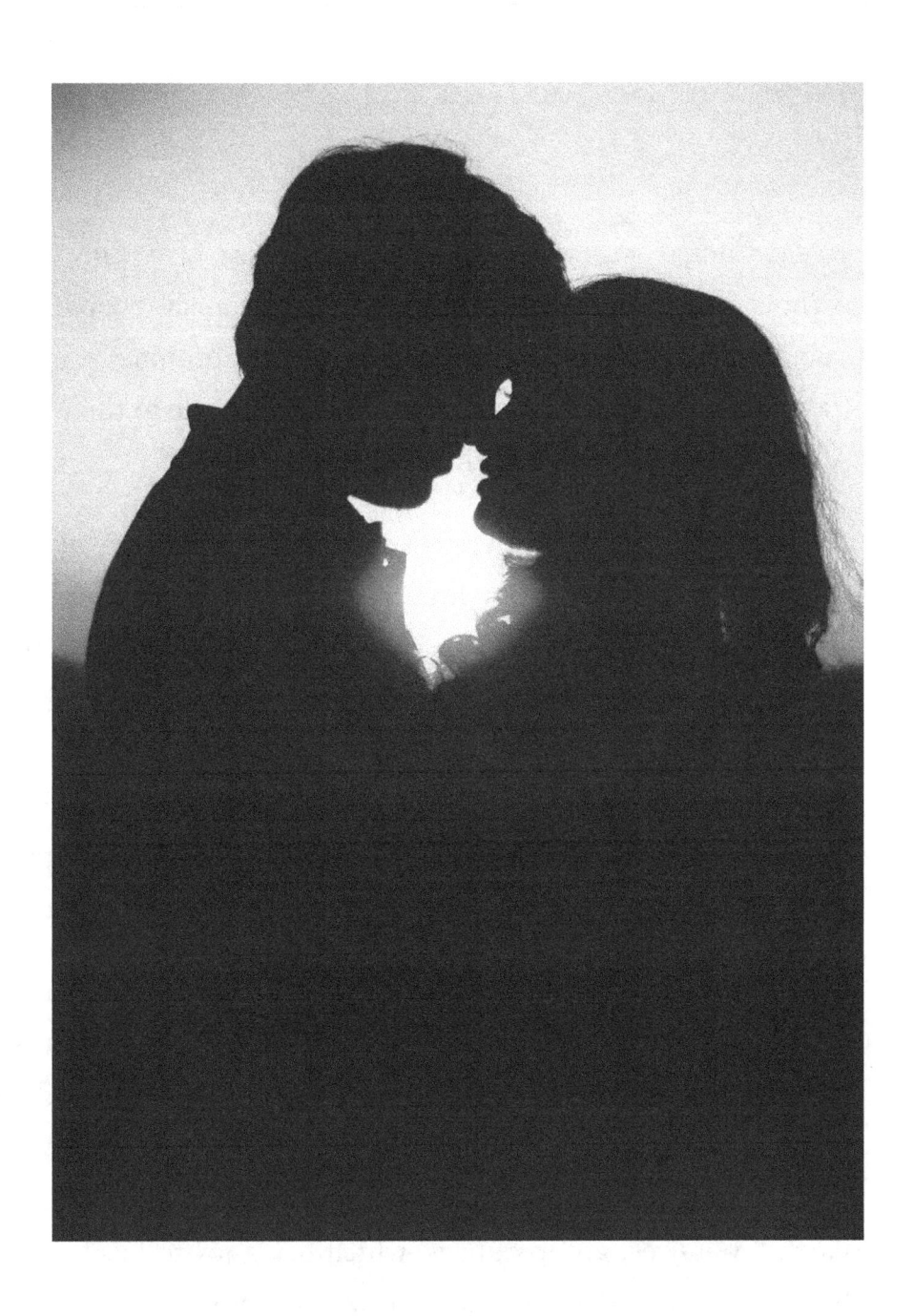

Conclusion

Hygge means enjoying life without stress. Live fully today without anguishing for tomorrow. The Danish people have managed to perfect this lifestyle in an extraordinary way and today they can boast of being the "happiest people in the world". And you?! Be inspired by Danish philosophy!

Turn your life into something you really love with Hygge! Some of the simplest moments are the most precious ones, stop chasing material goods. In this book you have learned how to be happy and healthy in your daily life, the secrets to making your life better, minimizing stress. You learned how to make your days more comforting. Above all, you learned not to focus hours on your smartphone, rather to create magical moments with the people you love.

Well... wonderful moments of sharing can change from city, to country, to nation! If we think of Italy, a coffee or a pizza with friends already makes us happy! England and Ireland are famous for sharing moments in the pub with friends after work. If we move to Spain or South America, there are so many parties, bonfires, group dances, which bring joy to local people. Behind the word Hygge there is a real social value, understood as collaboration, tolerance and sharing between individuals.

As you can see even if a word is missing, Hygge is everywhere! In conclusion we can say that the hyggelig moments are those moments, those moments that make you happy.

For this I want to greet you with a very hygge game: create your Hygge-word by putting the word "Hygge" or at the beginning or end of the sentence, example Hygge-Read of Magic, this new word indicates those beautiful moments that we spend together, talking about spiritual themes and our growth, sharing experiences with love and without judgment. Know that in general the Danes prefer to use Hygge as a prefix, therefore at the beginning of the word, but it could also be put at the end.

Now it's up to you to create your Hygge Paole, or Hygge-Reading you will see that by using them you will go and do things with a different spirit and with a whole hyggeling energy!

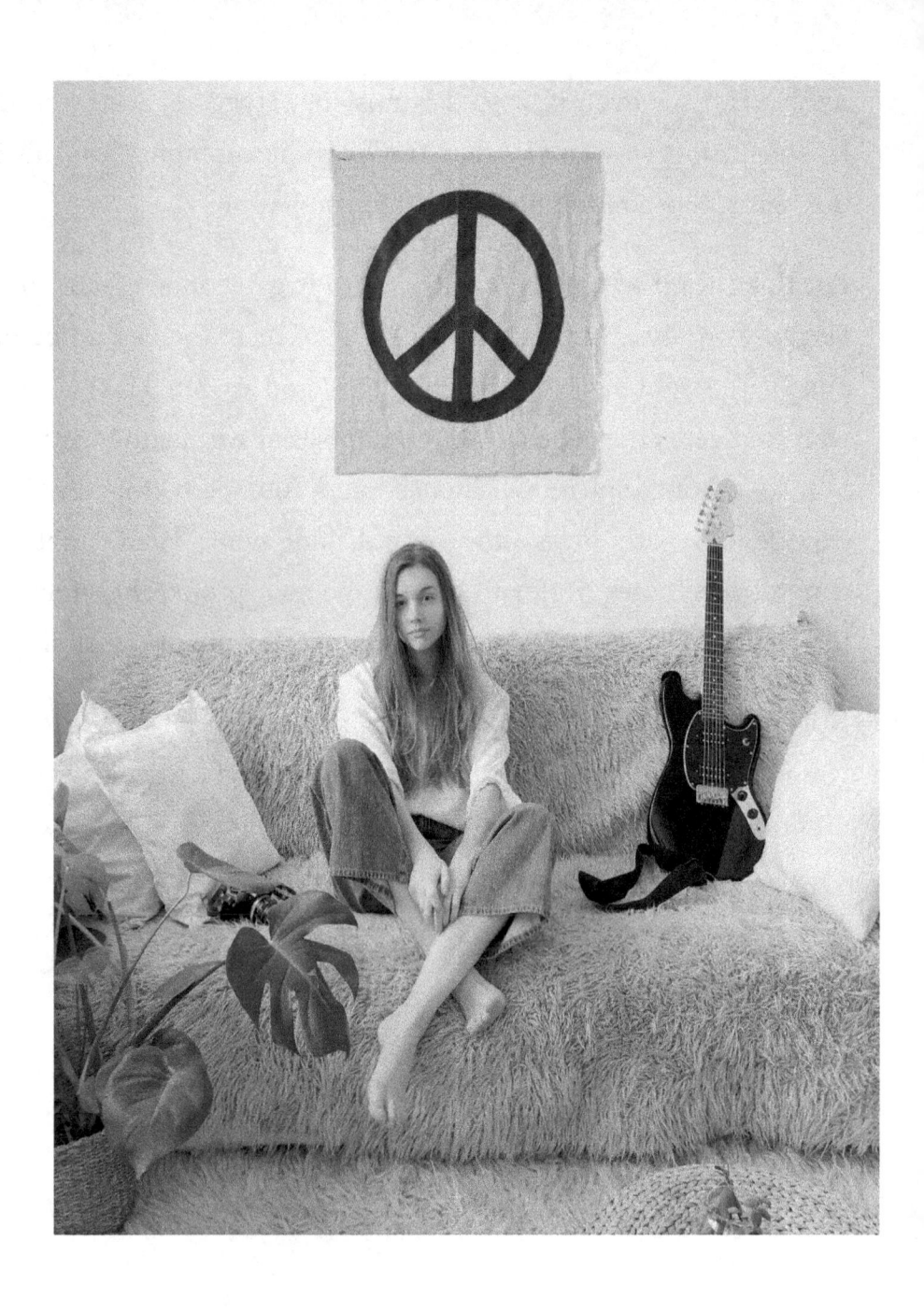

CPSIA information can be obtained
at www.ICGtesting.com
Printed in the USA
BVHW081955091120
592859BV00012B/1488